DORLAND'S DENTISTRY SPELLER

Consultant

RAYMOND J. FONSECA, DMD
Dean, University of Pennsylvania School of
  Dental Medicine
Philadelphia, Pennsylvania

Consultant for Syllabication

CAROL A. HART, PhD
Narberth, Pennsylvania

DORLAND'S DENTISTRY SPELLER

W.B. SAUNDERS COMPANY
A Division of Harcourt Brace & Company
Philadelphia London Toronto Montreal Sydney Tokyo

W.B. SAUNDERS COMPANY
A Division of
Harcourt Brace & Company

The Curtis Center
Independence Square West
Philadelphia, Pennsylvania 19106

Library of Congress Cataloging-in-Publication Data

Dorland's dentistry speller.

   p.   cm.

ISBN 0–7216–4572–0

1. Dentistry—Terminology.   I. W.B. Saunders Company.
   II. Title: Dentistry Speller.   [DNLM: 1. Dentistry—
   nomenclature.   WU 15 D711]

RK28.D67   1993

617.6′0014–dc20

DNLM/DLC   92–13389

DORLAND'S DENTISTRY SPELLER   ISBN 0–7216–4572–0

Printed in the United States of America.

Last digit is the print number: 9   8   7   6   5   4   3   2   1

Preface

With the publication of this volume, *Dorland's Dentistry Speller* joins the line of medical specialty spellers founded on the *Dorland's Illustrated Medical Dictionary* database. This book contains a comprehensive list of terms used in the dental specialties, as well as those used in oral and maxillofacial surgery. As in previous spellers, hard to find terms have been given multiple listings in order to make the book easier to use; an eponymic term, for example, will be found not only at the common noun but also at each of the eponyms. A system of acceptable end of line breaks has also been included.

The word list has been derived from a variety of sources, including the database for *Dorland's Illustrated Medical Dictionary*. Also included among the sources are texts, monographs, and journals and specialty dictionaries and references. Special attention has been devoted to difficult terms such as eponyms and trademarks, and Latin terminology has received full coverage.

We are very grateful to Raymond J. Fonseca, DMD, who thoroughly reviewed the terms list, and to Carol A. Hart, PhD, who provided the syllabication of the main entries. Thanks are also due to Gabriel Fonseca for his valuable assistance. Their efforts have been extremely helpful in ensuring the authoritativeness and comprehensiveness of *Dorland's Dentistry Speller*.

DOUGLAS M. ANDERSON
Chief Lexicographer

How This Book Is Arranged

Order of Entries

Dorland's Dentistry Speller follows the same scheme of arrangement as *Dorland's Illustrated Medical Dictionary*. Main entries follow one another in letter-by-letter alphabetical order regardless of spaces or hyphens that occur within them; compound entries consisting of one or more adjectives and a noun will be found as subentries under the noun. In some cases where there might be a question about where to look to find an entry, entries have been given in more than one place, even under an adjective.

Eponymic terms. Terms containing a proper name are given multiple listings, once under the thing named and once under each eponym. Thus *Hallermann-Streiff syndrome* is listed as:

> syndrome
>   Hallermann-Streiff s.
>
> Hallermann
>   H.-Streiff syndrome
>
> Streiff
>   Hallermann-S. syndrome

Umlauts are ignored for alphabetization, and proper names beginning *Mc* or *Mac* are alphabetized as though spelled *Mac*.

Subentries

Each subentry appears on a new line following the main entry and is indented. The main entry word in a subentry is represented only by the initial letter (as *Tomes f.* under *fiber*), with three exceptions. For regular English plurals, the abbreviation is the initial letter followed by *'s* (as *gingival f's* under *fiber*). For irregular or Greek or Latin plurals, the entire plural form is written out (as *dentes permanentes* under *dens*). For possessive forms, the initial letter is followed by *'s* (as *M's teeth* for *Moon's teeth*). In subentries the main entry word is ignored for alphabetization, as are prepositions, conjunctions, and articles.

Possessive Forms

The use of the possessive in eponyms is controversial. This book follows the example of *Dorland's Illustrated Medical Dictionary*, that is, the *'s* is favored where the sources for a term justify its appearance. Whether or not to use the possessive form is a matter left to the individual; owing to the present lack of consistency and consensus, no prescription can be given.

Abbreviations and Acronyms

A number of abbreviations and acronyms are given, together with the words or phrases that they stand for. The selection is of course only a small fraction of the abbreviations and acronyms in actual use. If more than one word or phrase is listed with an abbreviation, the terms are given in alphabetical order and each additional term is placed on a new line and indented.

Word Divisions

Acceptable word divisions are given for main entries; syllabication is based on pronunciation. Not all syllable breaks are shown; for example, because single letters at the beginnings and ends of words may not be separated from the rest of the word, such divisions are not given. Likewise, single letters should not be separated from the word elements they belong to in compound words. Breaks that could confuse the reader as to the meaning of a word are to be avoided. In many cases, words may be broken at other places than the ones that appear in this book (for example, different pronunciations imply different word breaks); it is impossible to show every break that could occur for every word. What appears here is one possible system.

Alternative Spellings

A number of works have alternative spellings, ranging from the difference of a single letter to the use of variant forms of Greek and Latin stems. Although every effort has been made to ensure that the spellings included in this book are valid, no indications of preference are given.

Brackets and Parentheses

Some entries require a bit of explanation; these explanations are enclosed in parentheses. Brackets are sometimes used as a part of Latin anatomical nomenclature to enclose an eponym in the genitive case; in this book such eponyms generally appear all lower case (as in *Dorland's Illustrated Medical Dictionary*), but an initial capital for the name is acceptable.

Plurals

Plurals for foreign words, nearly all of them Greek and Latin, are given with the appropriate entries. In addition, they are given again as separate entries if they do not occur within a few lines of the singular form.

Contents

AAA (autolyzed antigen-
  extracted allogeneic) bone

AACD
  American Academy of
  Cosmetic Dentistry

AADE
  American Association of
  Dental Editors
  American Association of
  Dental Examiners

AADGP
  American Academy of
  Dental Group Practice

AADP
  American Academy of
  Dental Prosthetics

AADPA
  American Academy of
  Dental Practice
  Administration

AADR
  American Academy of
  Dental Radiology

AADS
  American Association of
  Dental Schools

AAE
  American Association of
  Endodontists

AAGFO
  American Academy of Gold
  Foil Operators

AAGO
  American Academy of
  Gnathologic Orthopedics

AAHD
  American Association of
  Hospital Dentists

AAID
  American Academy of
  Implant Dentistry

AAMP
  American Academy of
  Maxillofacial Prosthetics

AAMRL
  American Association of
  Medical Records
  Librarians

AAO
  American Association of
  Orthodontists

AAOGP
  American Academy of
  Orthodontics for the
  General Practitioner

AAOM
  American Academy of Oral
  Medicine

AAOMS
  American Association of
  Oral and Maxillofacial
  Surgeons

AAOP
  American Academy of Oral
  Pathology

AAP
  American Academy of
  Pedodontics
  American Academy of
  Periodontology

AAPHD
  American Association of
  Public Health Dentists

Aar·skog
  A. syndrome

Aase
  A. syndrome

Abbe
  A.-Estlander flap

Ab·bot
  A's paste

ABC
  Air Barrier Coating

ABE
  American Board of
    Endodontics

Abell
  A. pliers

ab·la·tion

ab·nor·mal·i·ty
  dental a.
  dentofacial a.
  eugnathic a.
  eugnathic dental a.
  mandibular a's
  maxillofacial a.

ABO
  American Board of
    Orthodontics

ABOMS
  American Board of Oral
    and Maxillofacial Surgery

ABOP
  American Board of Oral
    Pathology

ABP
  American Board of
    Pedodontics
  American Board of
    Periodontology
  American Board of
    Prosthodontics

abrade

abra·sion
  betel nut a.
  bobby pin a.
  dental a.
  dentifrice a.
  denture a.

abra·sion *(continued)*
  a. of gingiva
  gingival a.
  occupational a.
  tobacco a.

abra·sive

abra·sor

ab·scess
  acute alveolar a.
  acute apical a.
  acute dentoalveolar a.
  acute periapical a.
  acute periodontal
    infrabony a.
  alveolar a.
  apical a.
  apical a., acute
  apical a., chronic
  Bezold's a.
  bicameral a.
  chronic apical a.
  chronic dentoalveolar a.
  chronic periapical a.
  chronic periodontal
    infrabony a.
  collar-button a.
  cornual a.
  dental a.
  dentoalveolar a.
  gingival a.
  internal Bezold's a.
  interradicular a.
  intramastoid a.
  lateral a.
  lateral alveolar a.
  mastoid a.
  odontogenic a.
  palatal a.
  parietal a.
  periapical a.
  pericoronal a.
  peridental a.
  periodontal a.
  phoenix a.
  pulp a.
  pulpal a.

ab·scess *(continued)*
    radicular a.
    shirt-stud a.

ab·strac·tion

abut·ment
    auxiliary a.
    implant a.
    intermediate a.
    isolated a.
    multiple a.
    PME a.
    primary a.
    secondary a.
    terminal a.

Acad·e·my of Den·tist·ry for the Hand·i·capped

Acad·e·my of Den·tist·ry In·ter·na·tion·al

Acad·e·my of Gen·er·al Den·tist·ry

Acad·e·my of Op·er·a·tive Den·tist·ry

Acad·e·my of Oral Dy·nam·ics

Acad·e·my of Os·seo·in·te·gra·tion

ac·an·tho·sis
    a. nigricans

Ac·cept·ed Den·tal Ther·a·peu·tics

ac·cep·tor
    hydrogen a.
    oxygen a.

ac·ces·so·ry

Ac·coe im·pres·sion ma·te·ri·al

Ac·coe tray ma·te·ri·al

Ac·cu Film ar·tic·u·lat·ing film

Ac·cu-Plac·er

Ac·cu·tane

ac·e·tyl·sal·i·cyl·ic acid

achon·dro·gen·e·sis
    a. type II

achon·dro·pla·sia

Ach·ro·my·cin V cap·sules

ac·id
    acetylsalicylic a.
    aminocaproic a.
    cellulosic a.
    polyacrylic a.
    polylactic a.
    poly-(L-lactic) a.
    tranexamic a.

acin·ic

Ac·ker·man
    A.-Proffit classification (for malocclusion)

Ac·ker·mann
    A. bar joint

aclu·sion

Ac·me ar·tic·u·la·tor

ACORDE
    A Consortium on Restorative Dentistry Education

ACORDE bur

ACP
    American College of Prosthodontists

ACPA
    American Cleft Palate Association

ac·quired im·mu·no·de·fi·cien·cy syn·drome (AIDS)

Ac·ri-Dense 3 pneu·mat·ic cur·ing unit

Ac·ri·lus·tre Pol·ish

ac·ro·dy·so·sto·sis

ac·ro·meg·a·ly

acryl·ic
Flexacryl rebase a.

ac·tin·ic

Ac·tino·ba·cil·lus
A. *actinomycetemcomitans*

Ac·ti·no·my·ces
A. *israelii*
A. *naeslundii*
A. *odontolyticus*
A. *propionica*
A. *viscosus*

ac·ti·no·my·co·sis
cervicofacial a.

ac·ti·va·tion

ac·ti·va·tor
Andresen a.
a. appliance
bow a.
functional a.
Harvold a.
Klammt a.
monoblock a.
open a.
Schwarz a.
Woodside a.

acu·mi·na·tum

ADA
American Dental
Association

ADAA
American Dental
Assistants Association

ADA Health Foun·da·tion Re·
search In·sti·tute

ad·a·man·tine

ad·a·man·ti·no·blas·to·ma

ad·a·man·ti·no·ma
a. polycysticum

ad·a·man·to·blast

ad·a·man·to·blas·to·ma
adenoid a.

ad·a·man·to·ma

ad·a·man·to-odon·to·ma

ad·a·mas
a. dentis

Ad·ams
A. clasps
A.-Oliver syndrome
A. suspension

ADA pro·ce·dure num·bers

ad·ap·ta·tion
masticatory a.

adap·ter
band a.

Adap·tic II com·pos·ite res·in

Adap·tic den·tal re·stor·ative

Adap·tol im·pres·sion ma·te·
ri·al

Adap·tol ther·mo·plas·tic im·
pres·sion ma·te·ri·al

ADA Uni·form Code on Den·
tal Pro·ce·dures and No·
men·cla·ture

Ad·di·son
A's disease

ad·e·no·am·e·lo·blas·
to·ma

ad·e·no·car·ci·no·ma
acinar cell a.
acinic cell a.
basal cell a.
low-grade papillary a.
polymorphous a.
polymorphous low-grade a.
terminal duct a.
terminal-duct papillary a.

ad·e·noid·ec·to·my

ad·e·no·ma
  a. adamantinum
  carcinoma ex pleomorphic
    a.
  monomorphic a.
  pleomorphic a.

ad·e·no·ma·toid

ad·e·no·ma·to·sis
  a. oris

Ad·er·er
  A. pliers

Ad·er·er No. 3 Bridge Gold

Ad·er·er "C" bridge

Ad·er·er No. 20 clasp

ad·he·sion

ad·he·sive
  dental a.
  denture a.
  Maryland bridge a.
  Panavia dental A.
  a. powder
  Scotchbond dental a.

ad·just·ment
  incisal guide a.
  occlusal a.
  postretention a.

ad·min·is·tra·tion
  practice a.

adre·no·cor·ti·coid

Ad·son
  A. forceps
  A.-Brown forceps

ad·vance·ment
  geniotomy a.
  Le Fort I maxillary a.
  Le Fort III midface a.
  mandibular a.
  maxillary a.
  maxillomandibular a.

Aeby
  A's muscle

aer·odon·tal·gia

aer·odon·tics

aero-odon·tal·gia

aero-odon·to·dy·nia

age
  dental a.
  a. hardening

agen·e·sis
  salivary gland a.

agent
  bleaching a.
  cavity lining a.
  disclosing a.
  glazing a.
  Heliobond bonding a.
  iodine disclosing a.
  Isolit wax release a.
  model release a.
  non-steroidal anti-
    inflammatory a's
    (NSAIA)
  Ora5 oral antibacterial a.
  polishing a.
  Pulpdent pulp capping a.
  silane coupling a.
  Superoxol bleaching a.
  Triad VLC bonding a.
  wetting a.

aglos·sia

ag·na·thia

ag·om·phi·a·sis

agom·phi·ous

ag·om·pho·sis

agran·u·lo·cy·to·sis

AH26 res·in

aid
  prosthetic speech a.

AIDS
  acquired immune
    deficiency syndrome

Air Bar·ri·er Coat·ing (ABC)

Air·bra·sive

air·way
    nasopharyngeal a.
    trumpeted nasal a's

AJCC
    American Joint Committee
        on Cancer

Aki·no·si
    A. technique

ala

al·ba

Al·bi·nus
    A. muscle

Al·bright
    A. hereditary
        osteodystrophy

Ale·co gold al·loy

Ale·co No. 4 gold al·loy

Ale·co No. 5 gold al·loy

Ale·co No. 9 gold al·loy

Al·ex·an·der
    A. attachment

al·fen·ta·nil

Al·gi·dent im·pres·sion ma·te·
    ri·al

al·gi·nate
    CutterJel a.

al·i·flu·rane

align·ment

Alike res·in

aline·ment

aliz·a·rin
    a. No. 6

Al·ka·lin·er cal·ci·um hy·drox·
    ide ma·te·ri·al

All-Bond 2 bond·ing sys·tem

All-Bond 2 Den·tal Adhesive
    Sys·tem

All·ce·zon base plate wax

Al·len
    A. periosteal elevator
    A's root pliers

All-Etch

Al·lis
    A. tissue forceps

Al·li·son
    A. forceps

al·lo·graft
    frozen a's

al·lo·plast

al·lo·plas·tic

al·lot·ri·odon·tia

al·loy
    a. A
    a. aging
    Aleco gold a.
    Aleco No. 4 gold a.
    Aleco No. 5 gold a.
    Aleco No. 9 gold a.
    amalgam a.
    Aristaloy a.
    Aristaloy CR a.
    a. B
    Artalloy a.
    Artalloy amalgam a.
    Balanced a.
    base metal crown and
        bridge a's
    Bean's a.
    Bridge III-C gold a.
    Bridge Partial IV-D gold a.
    Caulk spherical a.
    chrome-cobalt a.
    chromium base casting a.
    chromium-cobalt-nickel
        base a.
    cobalt-chromium a.
    Contour a.
    Crown No. 1 gold a.

al·loy *(continued)*
- Crown No. 3 gold a.
- Crown Hylastic gold a.
- Crown Knapp No. 3 gold a.
- Crown Supreme gold a.
- Crown TT gold a.
- cut a.
- cut amalgam a.
- a. D
- Dee-Eighteen gold a.
- Deeone gold a.
- Deepep-Hard gold a.
- Deesix gold a.
- Deetwo gold a.
- dental a.
- dental amalgam a.
- dental casting gold a.
- a. E
- Dispersalloy a.
- Duralloy a.
- Eclipse a.
- a. F
- Firmilay a.
- Forticast a.
- gold a.
- gold-copper a.
- a. HS21
- a. HS31
- Image a.
- Ionosphere a.
- JD a.
- Jelenko No. 7 gold a.
- Jel-Span a.
- LG a.
- Liberty a.
- Linc a.
- low silver a.
- Luxalloy a.
- Majority a.
- mercury a.
- a.-mercury ratio
- Miracast a.
- mixed type a.
- Modulay a.
- Monogram II a.
- Monogram III a.
- Mowrey 695 amalgam a.
- Mowrey 120 gold a.

al·loy *(continued)*
- Mowrey No. 8 gold a.
- Mowrey S-1 gold a.
- Mowrey S-3 gold a.
- Ney-Oro a.
- Nobillium a.
- Olympia a.
- Optaloy a.
- Option a.
- Perma-Bond a.
- Platinore a.
- preamalgamated a.
- Royal a.
- Shofu spherical a.
- silver-copper a.
- Silver Crest a.
- silver-palladium a.
- silver-tin a.
- solid solution a.
- spherical amalgam a.
- stellite a.
- Sterngold 1 gold a.
- Sterngold 2 gold a.
- Sterngold 3 gold a.
- Sterngold 5 gold a.
- Sterngold B gold a.
- Sterngold G-43 noble metal a.
- Sterngold S gold a.
- Sterngold Supercast gold a.
- Stratosphere a.
- Sturdicast a.
- Suncast a.
- Suteraloy amalgam a.
- Sybraloy a.
- tin-antimony a.
- Troposphere a.
- Tytin a.
- UltraGold a.
- Unison a.
- Valiant a.
- Valiant Ph.D. a.
- Valiant Snap-Set a.
- Velvalloy amalgam a.
- Vitallium a.
- zinc-free a.

al·loy·age

alu·mi·num
    a. oxide
    a. phosphate
    a. sulfate

Alu·wax

Al·veo·form

Al·veo·graf

al·veo·lal·gia

al·ve·o·lar

al·ve·o·late

al·ve·o·lec·to·my
    transeptal a.

al·ve·o·li·tis
    a. sicca dolorosa

al·ve·o·lo·cla·sia

al·ve·o·lo·con·dy·lar

al·ve·o·lo·den·tal

al·ve·o·lo·la·bi·al

al·ve·o·lo·lin·gual

al·ve·o·lo·me·rot·o·my

al·ve·o·lo·na·sal

al·ve·o·lo·pal·a·tal

al·ve·o·lo·plas·ty
    interradicular a.
    intraseptal a.

al·ve·o·lot·o·my

al·ve·o·lus *pl.* al·ve·o·li
    buccal a.
    canine a.
    dental a.
    a. dentalis
    alveoli dentales
      mandibulae
    alveoli dentales maxillae
    distobuccal a.
    first premolar a.
    lingual a.
    maxillary first molar a.

al·ve·o·lus *(continued)*
    mesiobuccal a.
    mucous a.
    salivary gland a.
    second premolar a.
    serous a.

Al·vo·gyl Dress·ing

amal·gam
    a. alloy
    a. condensation
    copper a.
    cut a. alloy
    dental a.
    gold a.
    a. mixer
    Mowrey 695 a. alloy
    pinned a.
    pin-retained a.
    pin-supported a.
    retrograde a.
    scrap a.
    silver a.
    spherical a. alloy

amal·gam·able

amal·ga·mate

amal·ga·ma·tion

amal·ga·ma·tor
    Crown a.
    Dentomat 3 a.
    Duomat 3 a.
    HS-1 a.
    Vari-Mix III a.
    Wig-L-Bug a.

Amal·gam Bond bond·ing sys·tem

am·bros·te·rol

amel·i·fi·ca·tion

amelo·blast

amelo·blas·tic

amelo·blas·to·ma
    acanthomatous a.
    basal cell a.

amelo·blas·to·ma *(continued)*
    calcifying a.
    cystic a.
    desmoplastic a.
    extraosseous a.
    extraosseous peripheral a.
    follicular a.
    granular cell a.
    multicystic a.
    peripheral a.
    malignant a.
    plexiform a.
    plexiform multicystic a.
    plexiform unicystic a.
    solid a.
    spindle a.
    uncommon a. with
      calcifications
    unicystic a.

amelo·den·ti·nal

amelo·gen·e·sis
    a. imperfecta

am·e·lo·gen·ic

am·e·lo·gen·in

Amer·i·can Acad·e·my of Cos·met·ic Den·tist·ry

Amer·i·can Acad·e·my of Den·tal Group Prac·tice

Amer·i·can Acad·e·my of Den·tal Prac·tice Ad·min·is·tra·tion

Amer·i·can Acad·e·my of Den·tal Ra·di·ol·o·gy

Amer·i·can Acad·e·my of Gna·tho·log·ic Or·tho·pe·dics

Amer·i·can Acad·e·my of Gold Foil Op·er·a·tors

Amer·i·can Acad·e·my of Im·plant Den·tist·ry

Amer·i·can Acad·e·my of Max·il·lo·fa·cial Pros·thet·ics

Amer·i·can Acad·e·my of Oral Med·i·cine

Amer·i·can Acad·e·my of Oral Pa·thol·o·gy

Amer·i·can Acad·e·my of Or·tho·don·tics for the Gen·er·al Prac·ti·tion·er

Amer·i·can Acad·e·my of Pe·do·don·tics

Amer·i·can Acad·e·my of Peri·odon·tol·o·gy

Amer·i·can As·so·ci·a·tion of Den·tal Ed·i·tors

Amer·i·can As·so·ci·a·tion of Den·tal Schools

Amer·i·can As·so·ci·a·tion of Hos·pi·tal Den·tists

Amer·i·can As·so·ci·a·tion of Oral and Max·il·lo·fa·cial Sur·geons

Amer·i·can As·so·ci·a·tion of Or·tho·don·tists

Amer·i·can As·so·ci·a·tion of Pub·lic Health Den·tists

Amer·i·can Board of Den·tal Pub·lic Health

Amer·i·can Board of En·do·don·tics

Amer·i·can Board of Oral and Max·il·lo·fa·cial Sur·gery

Amer·i·can Board of Oral Pa·thol·o·gy

Amer·i·can Board of Oral Sur·gery

Amer·i·can Board of Or·tho·don·tics

Amer·i·can Board of Pe·do·don·tics

Amer·i·can Board of Peri·odon·tol·o·gy

Amer·i·can Board of Pros·tho·don·tics

Amer·i·can Cleft Pal·ate As·so·ci·a·tion

Amer·i·can Cleft Pal·ate As·so·ci·a·tion clas·si·fi·ca·tion

Amer·i·can Col·lege of Den·tists

Amer·i·can Col·lege of Oral and Max·il·lo·fa·cial Sur·geons

Amer·i·can Col·lege of Pros·tho·don·tists

Amer·i·can Col·lege of Sur·geons

Amer·i·can Den·tal As·sis·tants As·so·ci·a·tion

Amer·i·can Den·tal As·so·ci·a·tion

Amer·i·can Den·tal As·so·ci·a·tion Health Foun·da·tion

Amer·i·can Den·tal As·so·ci·a·tion Uni·form Code on Den·tal Pro·ce·dures and No·men·cla·ture

Amer·i·can Den·tal Hy·gien·ists' As·so·ci·a·tion

Amer·i·can Fund for Den·tal Health

Amer·i·can Gold "B" Bridge

Amer·i·can Gold "C" Par·tial Ex·tra Hard

Amer·i·can Gold "M-H" In·lay

Amer·i·can Gold "M" In·lay Me·di·um

Amer·i·can Gold "T" Bridge Hard

Amer·i·can Joint Com·mit·tee on Can·cer

Amer·i·can Na·tion·al Stan·dards Com·mit·tee MD156 for Den·tal Ma·te·ri·als and De·vices

Ames plas·tic por·ce·lain

ami·no·ca·pro·ic acid

ami·no·gly·co·side

am·i·noph·yl·line

ami·o·da·rone

AML
    acute myelogenous leukemia

amox·i·cil·lin

Amox·il

am·pho·ter·i·cin B

amp·i·cil·lin

am·pu·ta·tion
    pulp a.
    root a.

am·y·loi·do·sis

amyo·troph·ic

an·al·ge·sia
    patient-controlled a.

anal·y·sis *pl.* anal·y·ses
    bite a.
    cephalometric a.
    craniofacial a.
    Downs' a.
    facial a.
    Harvold a.
    occlusal a.
    Sassouni a.
    Steiner a.
    Wits a.

anat·o·my
    dental a.

An·be·sol

an·chor
   endosteal implant a.
   a. molar
   Zest implant a's

an·chor·age
   Baker a.
   cervical a.
   compound a.
   extramaxillary a.
   extraoral a.
   intermaxillary a.
   intraoral a.
   maxillomandibular a.
   multiple a.
   occipital a.
   precision a.
   reciprocal a.
   reinforced a.
   simple a.
   stationary a.

An·der·son
   Roger-A. pin

An·dre·sen
   A. activator
   A. appliance
   A. monoblock appliance

An·drews
   A. bar
   A. bridge

An·dy Gump
   A.G. deformity

ane·mia
   aplastic a.
   iron deficiency a.
   pernicious a.
   sickle cell a.

an·es·the·sia
   electronic dental a. (EDA)
   lip a.
   local a.

an·eu·rysm
   false a.
   traumatic a.

an·eu·rys·mal

An·gel·man
   A. syndrome

an·gi·na
   Ludwig's a.

an·gio·ede·ma

an·gio·fi·bro·ma
   juvenile nasopharyngeal a.
   nasopharyngeal a.

an·gi·og·ra·phy

an·gio·my·o·ma

an·gio·sar·co·ma

An·gle
   A's band
   A's classification (for
      malocclusion)
   A's splint

an·gle
   a. of aberration
   alveolar profile a.
   anterior a. of petrous
      portion of temporal bone
   anterior inferior a. of
      sphenoid bone
   anterior superior a. of
      parietal bone
   a. of aperture
   axial a.
   axial line a.
   Bennett a.
   buccal a's
   bucco-occlusal line a.
   cavity a's
   cavosurface a.
   cephalic a.
   cephalometric a.
   chi a.
   condylar a.
   condylar a. of mandible
   a. of convexity
   cranial a.
   craniofacial a.
   critical a.

an·gle *(continued)*
cusp a.
cusp plane a.
Daubenton's a.
distal a's
distal incisal a.
distobucco-occlusal point a.
distolabial line a.
distolabioincisal point a.
distolingual line a.
distolinguoincisal point a.
distolinguo-occlusal point
   a.
disto-occlusal line a.
ethmocranial a.
ethmoid a.
facial a.
Frankfort-mandibular
   plane a.
frontal a. of parietal bone
gonial a.
horizontal a.
impedance a.
incisal a.
incisal guide a.
incisal mandibular plane
   a.
Jacquart's a.
a. of jaw
kappa a.
labial a's
labioincisal line a.
lateral a. of eye
limiting a.
line a.
lingual a's
linguoincisal line a.
linguo-occlusal line a.
a. of mandible
mandibular a.
mandibular profile a.
mastoid a. of parietal bone
maxillary a.
medial a. of eye
mesial a's
mesial incisal a.
mesiobuccal line a.
mesiolabial line a.

an·gle *(continued)*
mesiolabioincisal point a.
mesiolingual line a.
mesiolinguoincisal point a.
mesiolinguoocclusal point
   a.
mesioocclusal line a.
metafacial a.
a. of mouth
a. of Mulder
nasal profile a.
nasolabial a.
occipital a. of parietal bone
olfactive a.
olfactory a.
ophryospinal a.
orifacial a.
parietal a.
parietal a. of sphenoid
   bone
a. of petrous portion of
   temporal bone
point a.
a. of polarization
posterior inferior a. of
   parietal bone
posterior superior a. of
   parietal bone
prophy a.
prophylaxis a.
Quatrefage's a.
Ranke's a.
Rivet's a.
Serres' a.
somatosplanchnic a.
sphenoid a.
sphenoidal a.
sphenoidal a. of parietal
   bone
superior a. of petrous
   portion of temporal bone
target a.
tooth a's
Topinard's a.
total profile a.
venous a.
a. of Virchow
Vogt's a.

an·gle *(continued)*
    Weisbach's a.
    Welcher's a.

an·gu·lar

an·hy·dride
    silicic a.

an·iso·dont

an·ky·lo·glos·sia

an·ky·lo·sis *pl.* an·ky·lo·ses
    condylar a.
    a. of teeth
    TMJ a.

an·ky·lot·o·my

ANLL
    acute nonlymphocytic
        leukemia

an·neal

an·neal·ing
    metal a.

an·odon·tia

anom·a·lad
    Robin's a.
    Pierre Robin a.
    Sturge-Weber a.

anom·a·lous

anom·a·ly
    branchial cleft a.
    dental a.
    dentofacial a.
    dysgnathic a.
    eugnathic a.
    eugnathic dental a.

ANSI
    American National
        Standards Institute

an·tag·o·nist

an·tero·clu·sion

An·tho·ny
    Shea-A. antral balloon

an·ti·car·io·gen·ic

an·ti·car·i·ous

an·ti·flux

an·ti·gen
    squamous cell carcinoma a.

an·ti·odon·tal·gic

an·ti·si·al·a·gogue

Ant·ley
    A.-Bixler syndrome

ant·odon·tal·gic

an·tro·at·ti·cot·o·my

an·tro·buc·cal

an·tro·cele

an·tro·dyn·ia

an·tro·nal·gia

an·tro·na·sal

an·tro·scope

an·tros·co·py

an·tros·to·my

an·tro·tome

an·trot·o·my

an·tro·tym·pan·ic

an·tro·tym·pan·i·tis

an·trum
    a. of Highmore

an·xi·ol·y·sis

AO/ASIF
    AO Study Group for
        Internal Fixation

AO/ASIF con·dy·lar pros·the·
ses

AO/ASIF re·con·struc·tion
    plate

AO Stu·dy Group for In·ter·
nal Fix·a·tion

AOT
    adenomatoid odontogenic
        tumor

AO-THORP re·con·struc·tion
    sys·tem

AP
    anteroposterior

Apa·cer·am im·plant

Apap

ap·a·tite

Apert
    A's syndrome

ap·er·tog·na·thia

apex

apex·i·fi·ca·tion

apexi·graph

Apexo el·e·va·tor

apexo·gen·e·sis

apexo·graph

aph·tha *pl.* aph·thae

aph·thous

ap·i·cal

api·cec·to·my

ap·i·ces

ap·i·ci·tis

ap·i·co·ec·to·my
    impaction a.

ap·i·cos·to·my

apla·sia
    condylar a.
    enamel and dentin a.

APL den·tal stone

ap·nea
    obstructive sleep a.

apoph·y·sis *pl.* apoph·y·ses
    genial a.
    a. of Ingrassias
    pterygoid a.

ap·pa·rat·us *pl.* ap·pa·rat·us,
    ap·pa·rat·us·es
    attachment a.
    Bouisson a.
    masticatory a.

ap·pli·ance
    acrylic head a.
    acrylic resin and copper
        band a.
    activator a.
    active plate a.
    Andresen a.
    Andresen monoblock a.
    Begg a.
    Bimler a.
    Bowles multiphase a.
    Coffin a.
    craniofacial a.
    Crozat a.
    Denholz a.
    differential force a.
    E-arch a.
    edgewise a.
    expansion plate a.
    extraoral a.
    finger-sucking re-education
        a.
    fixed a.
    fracture a.
    Frankel a.
    functional a.
    Griffin a.
    Haas expansion a.
    habit-breaking a.
    Hawley a.
    hay rake a.
    Herbst a.
    hybrid functional a.
    jackscrew a.
    Jackson a.
    Johnston twin wire a.
    jumping-the-bite a.
    Kesling a.

ap·pli·ance *(continued)*
  Kingsley a.
  labiolingual a.
  light round-wire a.
  lingual a.
  lip habit a.
  Mayne muscle control a.
  monoblock a.
  mouthstick a.
  Mühlemann a.
  multibanded a.
  multiphase a.
  Nord a.
  obturator a.
  occlusal a.
  occlusal overlay a.
  orthodontic a.
  palatal expansion a.
  palatal obturator a.
  permanent a.
  pin and tube a.
  prosthetic a.
  regulating a.
  removable a.
  retaining a.
  ribbon arch a.
  rigid fixation a.
  Roger Anderson pin
    fixation a.
  Schwarz a.
  split plate a.
  straight-arch a.
  straight-wire a.
  Sved-type a.
  therapeutic a.
  thumb-sucking a.
  tongue-thrust a.
  twin wire a.
  unilateral fixed a.
  universal a.
  visceral deglutition a.
  visceral swallowing a.
  Walker a.
ap·pli·ca·tor
  Dr. Thompson's Color
    Transfer A's
  root canal a.

ap·po·si·tion
ap·proach
  buttonhole a.
  lingual a.
  Risdon a.
apron
  lead a.
APS
  American Prosthodontic
    Society
ap·ty·a·lia
ap·ty·a·lism
Aqua·fix ir·ri·gat·ing sy·ringes
arc
  adjustive a's of closure
  bregmatolambdoid a.
  a's of mandibular closure
  nasobregmatic a.
  naso-occipital a.
arch
  alveolar a.
  alveolar a. of mandible
  alveolar a. of maxilla
  a. bar
  basal a.
  bypass a.
  dental a.
  dental a., inferior
  dental a., superior
  depressing a.
  edentulous a.
  glossopalatine a.
  Gothic a. tracing
  horseshoe-shaped a.
  inferior dental a.
  intrusion a.
  labial a.
  labial and lingual a's
  leveling a.
  lingual a.
  lingual a., fixed
  lingual a., fixed-removable
  lingual a., passive
  lingual a., stationary

arch *(continued)*
    lingual holding a.
    malar a.
    mandibular a.
    maxillary a.
    Mershon a.
    Nance holding a.
    oral a.
    palatal a.
    palatine a., anterior
    palatine a., posterior
    palatoglossal a.
    palatomaxillary a.
    palatopharyngeal a.
    palpebral a., inferior
    partially edentulous a.
    passive lingual a.
    residual a.
    residual dental a.
    ribbon a.
    square a.
    stationary lingual a.
    superior dental a.
    tapering a.
    trapezoidal a.
    V-shaped a.
    W a.
    a. width
    zygomatic a.

arch·wire
    beta-titanium a.
    copper a.
    labial a.
    nickel-titanium a.
    preformed a.
    rectangular a.
    stainless steel a.

ar·cus *pl.* ar·cus
    a. alveolaris mandibulae
    a. alveolaris maxillae
    a. dentalis inferior
    a. dentalis superior
    a. palatini

ar·ea *pl.* ar·eae, ar·eas
    basal seat a.
    bilaminar a. of articular
      disk

ar·ea *(continued)*
    contact a.
    denture-bearing a.
    denture foundation a.
    denture-supporting a.
    hypoglossal a.
    a. hypoglossi
    impression a.
    interglobular a's
    interproximal contact a.
    pear-shaped a.
    post dam a.
    posterior palatal seal a.
    postpalatal seal a.
    pressure a.
    recipient a.
    relief a.
    rest a.
    retention a. of tooth
    retromolar a.
    retromylohyoid a.
    rugae a.
    saddle a.
    self-cleansing a.
    stress-bearing a.
    stress-supporting a.
    supporting a.

Aris·ta·loy al·loy

Aris·ta·loy CR al·loy

Ar·kan·sas stone

arm
    bar clasp a.
    circumferential clasp a.
    endosteal implant a.
    engine a.
    reciprocal a.
    retensive a.
    retention a.
    retentive a.
    retentive circumferential
      clasp a.
    stabilizing a.
    stabilizing circumferential
      clasp a.
    T clasp a.
    Y clasp a.

ar·ma·men·tar·i·um
    endodontic a.
    periodontal a.

Ar·nett-TMP ri·gid fix·a·tion
    sys·tem

ar·range·ment
    anterior tooth a.
    tooth a.

Ar·tal·loy al·loy

Ar·tal·loy amal·gam al·loy

ar·te·ria *pl.* ar·te·riae
    arteriae alveolares
      superiores anteriores
    a. alveolaris inferior
    a. alveolaris superior
      posterior
    a. labialis inferior
    a. labialis superior
    a. lingualis
    a. masseterica
    a. maxillaris
    a. mentalis
    a. palatina ascendens
    a. palatina descendens
    a. palatina major
    arteriae palatinae minores
    a. pharyngea ascendens
    a. profunda linguae
    a. sublingualis
    a. submentalis

ar·te·ri·og·ra·phy

ar·te·ri·o·la *pl.* ar·te·ri·o·lae

ar·te·ri·ole

ar·te·rio·ve·nous

ar·ter·itis *pl.* ar·ter·it·i·des
    temporal a.

ar·te·ry
    angular a.
    anterior dental a's
    anterior inferior cerebellar
      a.

ar·te·ry *(continued)*
    anterior superior alveolar
      a's
    articular a.
    ascending palatine a.
    basilar a.
    buccal a.
    buccinator a.
    carotid a.
    deep lingual a.
    descending palatine a.
    dorsal lingual a's
    ethmoid a.
    facial a.
    greater palatine a.
    inferior alveolar a.
    inferior dental a.
    inferior labial a.
    interdental a's
    interradicular a's
    labyrinthine a.
    lesser palatine a's
    lingual a.
    major palatine a.
    mandibular a.
    masseteric a.
    maxillary a.
    mental a.
    minor palatine a's
    mylohyoid a.
    perforating alveolar a's
    pharyngeal a., ascending
    pontine a's
    posterior cerebral a.
    sublingual a.
    submental a.
    superior cerebellar a.
    superior dental a.
    superior labial a.

ar·thral·gia

ar·thri·tis *pl.* ar·thrit·i·des
    condylar a.
    hypertrophic a.
    infectious a. of
      temporomandibular joint
    pseudorheumatoid a.

ar·thri·tis *(continued)*
    traumatic a. of
      temporomandibular joint

ar·throg·ra·phy
    anteroposterior (AP) a.

ar·throl·y·sis

ar·throp·a·thy
    psoriatic a.

ar·thro·plas·ty
    interposition a.
    intracapsular
      temporomandibular joint
      a.

ar·thro·scope
    ultrathin a.

ar·thros·copy
    temporomandibular joint
      (TMJ) a.

ar·thro·sis

ar·thro·to·mog·ra·phy
    dual space AP a.

ar·throt·o·my
    open a.

Ar·ti·co·dent ar·tic·u·lat·ing
    pa·per

Ar·ti·cu-Film ar·tic·u·lat·ing
    film

ar·tic·u·lar

ar·tic·u·la·re

ar·tic·u·late

ar·tic·u·lat·ed

ar·tic·u·la·tio *pl.* ar·tic·u·la·
    ti·o·nes
    a. dentoalveolaris
    a. mandibularis

ar·tic·u·la·tion
    articulator a.
    balanced a.
    ball-and-socket a.

ar·tic·u·la·tion *(continued)*
    composite a.
    compound a.
    dental a.
    dentoalveolar a.
    gliding a.
    mandibular a.
    manubriosternal a.
    maxillary a.
    mediocarpal a.
    temporomandibular a.
    temporomaxillary a.

ar·tic·u·la·tor
    Acme a.
    adjustable a.
    anatomic a.
    arcon a.
    Balkwell a.
    Bergström's a.
    Christensen a.
    Denar a.
    dental a.
    Dentatus a.
    Evans' a.
    Granger a.
    Gysi's a.
    Hanau a.
    Hanau 130-21 a.
    hinge a.
    Ney a.
    plain-line a.
    semiadjustable a.
    Walker a.
    Whip-Mix a.

Ar·ti-Spot sol·vent

as·bes·tos

ASC 52 at·tach·ment

Asch
    A. forceps
    A's splint

As·cher
    A's syndrome

ASPA ce·ment

as·per·gil·lo·sis

as·pi·ra·tion

as·pi·ra·tor
    dental a.
    Frazier a.

as·pi·rin

As·sé·zat
    A's triangle

as·sis·tant
    administrative dental a.
    Certified Dental A.
    chairside dental a.
    control dental a.
    coordinating a.
    coordinating dental a.
    currently certified dental
        a.
    dental a.
    expanded function dental
        a.
    extended function dental a.
    foil a.
    medical laboratory a.
    Registered Dental A.

as·so·ci·a·tion
    aniridia-Wilms tumor a.
    CHARGE a.
    MURCS a.

astrin·gent

asym·me·try
    chin a.
    facial a.
    maxillary a.
    midline a.
    unilateral a.

At·a·rax

ate·los·teo·gen·e·sis

aten·o·lol

At·i·van

at·lan·to·oc·cip·i·tal

at·loi·do·oc·cip·i·tal

At·ra·loc nee·dle

atroph·ic

at·ro·phied

at·ro·phy
    afunctional a.
    alveolar a.
    gingival a.
    hemifacial a.
    precocious advanced a.
    precocious advanced
        alveolar a.
    pulp a.
    reticular pulp a.

at·ro·pine

at·tach·ment
    abnormal frenulum a.
    abnormal frenum a.
    Alexander a.
    a. apparatus
    ASC 52 a.
    Ballard stress equalizer a.
    ball-and-socket a.
    band a.
    bar a.
    Bowles a.
    Bowles multiphase a.
    Ceka a.
    channel shoulder pin a.
    Chayes a.
    C & L a.
    Clark a.
    C & M 637 a.
    combined a.
    Conex a.
    Crismani a.
    Crismani combined a.
    CSP (crown shoulder pin)
        a.
    Cu-Sil a.
    Dalbo a.
    Dalbo extracoronal a.
    Dalbo stud a.
    Dalla Bona a.
    Dolder bar joint a.
    Dolder bar unit a.
    dovetail a.
    dowel rest a.

at·tach·ment *(continued)*
    edgewise a.
    epithelial a. (of Gottlieb)
    extracoronal a.
    friction a.
    gingival a.
    gingival a. (of Gottlieb)
    gingival latch a.
    Hade-Ring a.
    Hart-Dunn a.
    Hruska a.
    implant superstructure a.
    internal a.
    intracoronal a.
    Ipsoclip a.
    key-and-keyway a.
    labial a.
    McCollum a.
    multiphase a.
    Neurohr spring-lock a.
    new a.
    orthodontic a.
    parallel a.
    Pin-Dalbo a.
    pinledge a.
    precision a.
    Pressomatic a.
    projection a.
    ribbon arch a.
    Roach a.
    Rothermann a.
    Schatzmann a.
    Schubiger a.
    Scott a.
    semiprecision a.
    Sherer a.
    slotted a.
    Stabilex a.
    Steiger's a.
    Steiger-Boitel a.
    Stern a.
    Stern G/A a.
    Stern gingival latch a.
    Stern G/L a.
    Stern stress-breaker a.
    stress-breaker a.
    stud a.
    superstructure a.

at·tach·ment *(continued)*
    Tach-E-Z a.
    twin wire a.
    universal orthodontic a.
    Zest Anchor system a.

At·test bio·log·i·cal in·di·ca·tors

at·trac·tion

at·tri·tion

atyp·i·cal

aug·men·ta·tion
    alveolar ridge a.
    bone a.
    chin a.
    malar a.
    mandibular a.
    onlay facial a.

Aug·men·tin

au·ric·u·lo·tem·po·ral

Aus·tin
    A. retractor

au·to·clave

Au·to·Mix com·pu·ter·ized mix·ing sys·tem

Au·to·Mix mix·ing unit

au·to·trans·plant

aux·il·i·a·ry
    dental a.
    expanded duty dental a.
    expanded function dental a.
    torquing a.

Avi·tene (microfibrillar collagen)

AVM
    arteriovenous malformation

avul·sion
    tooth a.

awl
    Obwegeser a.
    Rowe zygomatic a.

ax·i·al

ax·io·buc·cal

ax·io·buc·co·cer·vi·cal

ax·io·buc·co·gin·gi·val

ax·io·buc·co·lin·gual

ax·io·cer·vi·cal

ax·io·dis·tal

ax·io·dis·to·cer·vi·cal

ax·io·dis·to·gin·gi·val

ax·io·dis·to·in·ci·sal

ax·io·dis·to-oc·clu·sal

ax·io·gin·gi·val

ax·i·og·ra·phy

ax·io·in·ci·sal

ax·io·la·bi·al

ax·io·la·bio·gin·gi·val

ax·io·la·bio·lin·gual

ax·io·lin·gual

ax·io·lin·guo·cer·vi·cal

ax·io·lin·guo·gin·gi·val

ax·io·lin·guo-oc·clu·sal

ax·io·me·si·al

ax·io·me·sio·cer·vi·cal

ax·io·me·sio·dis·tal

ax·io·me·sio·gin·gi·val

ax·io·me·sio·in·ci·sal

ax·io·me·sio-oc·clu·sal

ax·io-oc·clu·sal

ax·io·pul·pal

ax·ip·e·tal

ax·is *pl.* ax·es
    basibregmatic a.
    basicranial a.
    basifacial a.
    binauricular a.
    cephalocaudal a.
    condylar a.
    condyle a.
    craniofacial a.
    a. cylinder
    dorsoventral a.
    Downs' Y a.
    facial a.
    hinge a.
    horizontal a.
    long a. of body
    longitudinal a.
    mandibular a.
    mandibular intercondylar
      hinge a.
    opening a.
    a. of preparation
    sagittal a. of mandible
    thyroid a.
    transverse a.
    vertical a.
    Y a.

az·lo·cil·lin

B
Bolton point
bregma
point B

b
point B

Ba
basion

ba
basion

Bab·bitt
B. metal

ba·cam·pi·cil·lin

Bac·i·tra·cin oint·ment

back·ing
alloy b.

Bac·te·roi·des
B. asaccharolyticus
B. corporis
B. endodontalis
B. forsythus
B. fragilis
B. gingivalis
B. intermedius
B. loescheii
B. melaninogenicus

Bai·lyn
B's classification (for
partially edentulous
arches)

Ba·ka·mi·jam
B. flap

bake

Bake·lite

Ba·ker
B. anchorage
B. inlay
B. inlay, extra hard

Ba·ker (continued)
B. inlay, hard

bak·ing
high biscuit b.
low biscuit b.
medium biscuit b.

bal·ance
facial b.
occlusal b.

Bal·anced al·loy

Balk·well
B. articulator

ball
fatty b. of Bichat

Bal·lard
B. stress equalizer
(attachment)

bal·loon
antral b.
Shea-Anthony antral b.
sinus b.

Bal·ters
B. bionator

Ban·croft
B. equation

band
anchor b.
apron b.
canine b.
b's of Bungner
clamp b.
contoured b.
elastic b.
b's of Hunter-Schreger
matrix b.
molar b.
orthodontic b.
preformed b.
premolar b.

band *(continued)*
    rubber b.
    b's of Schreger
    stainless steel b.
    tension b.

ban·dage
    extraoral b.
    intraoral adhesive b.

ban·de·lette

band·ing
    full-mouth b.
    tension b.
    tooth b.

Bank·er
    B's sponge

ban·thine

bar
    Andrews b.
    anterior palatal b.
    arch b.
    beaded palatal b.
    buccal b.
    b. clasp
    connecting b.
    connector b.
    Dolder b.
    double lingual b.
    Erich arch b.
    fixable-removable cross
      arch b.
    fixed lingual b.
    Gaerny b.
    Gilson fixable-removable b.
    horseshoe b.
    I b.
    b. joint
    Kazanjian 122 b.
    Kennedy b.
    labial b.
    lingual b.
    mesostructure b.
    occlusal rest b.
    palatal b.
    Passavant's b.
    posterior palatal b.

bar *(continued)*
    primary b.
    RP-I b.
    secondary b.
    Steiger-Boitel b.
    T b. of Kazanjian

bar·bi·tur·ate

Bar·kann
    B's technique

Bar·ker
    B's point

Barn·hart
    B. curet

Bar·ri·caid VLC peri·odon·tal
wound dress·ing

Bar·ri·er den·tin con·di·tion·
er

Bar·ri·er den·tin seal·ant

Bar·tho·lin
    B's duct

ba·sad

ba·sal

base
    acrylic resin b.
    alar b.
    apical b.
    BaseLine glass ionomer b./
      liner
    cavity b.
    cement b.
    cheoplastic b.
    denture b.
    denture b., tinted
    Dropsin calcium hydroxide
      b.
    free-end extension b.
    intermediary b.
    metal b.
    plastic b.
    Preline b./liner
    Prisma VLC Dycal calcium
      hydroxide b.

base *(continued)*
    processed denture b.
    proximal cement b.
    record b.
    saddle denture b.
    shellac b's
    sprue b.
    stabilized b.
    strong b.
    temporary b.
    Timeline b./liner
    tinted denture b.
    tissue-supported b.
    tissue-tissue–supported b.
    tooth-borne b.
    trial b.
    Vitrebond b./liner
    weak b.

base·line

Base·Line glass ion·o·mer
  base/lin·er

base·plate
    gutta-percha b.
    b. material
    permanent b.
    stabilized b.

ba·si·hy·al

ba·si·hy·oid

ba·sio·glos·sus

Bass
    B. brush
    B. method of
      toothbrushing
    B. technique
    B. toothbrush

Bat·tle
    B's sign

Bau·dens
    B. wiring

Baum·gart·ner
    B. needle holder

Bay·si·lex Hy·dro·activ im·
  pres·sion ma·te·ri·al

Bay·si·lex im·pres·sion ma·te·
  ri·al

BBC
    Buffing Bar Compound

bead
    acrylic cement b's
    methylmethacrylate b's
    tobramycin-impregnated
      b's

Beals
    B. syndrome

beam
    cantilever b.
    central b.
    continuous b.
    b. deflection
    homogeneous b.
    monochromatic b.
    primary b.
    restrained b.
    simple b.
    useful b.

Bean
    B's alloy

bear·ing
    central b.

Beck·with
    B.-Wiedemann syndrome

bec·lo·meth·a·sone di·pro·pi·
  o·nate

Bec·o·nase

Bee·pen

Bee·ren·donk
    B. caliper

bees·wax

Begg
    B's appliance
    B. bracket
    B's technique
    B's theory
    B. uprighting spring

Beh·çet
    B's syndrome

Bell
    B's palsy

bend
    first order b's
    second order b's
    third order b's
    V b's

Ben·da Brush

Ben·e·fit den·ture ad·he·sive

Ben·nett
    B. angle
    B. movement

ben·zo·caine

Ben·zo·dent

ben·zo·di·az·e·pine

Ben·zo-jel

Berg·ström
    B's articulator

Ber·lin
    B's edema

Ber·nays
    B. sponge

be·ta·meth·a·sone

bev·el
    cavosurface b.
    contra b.
    instrument b.
    reverse b.
    standing b.
    under b.

Be·zold
    B's abscess

BHN
    Brinell hardness number

bi·bev·eled

bi·cus·pid

bi·cus·pi·dal

bi·cus·pi·date

bi·cus·poid

bi·den·tal

bi·den·tate

bi·fid

bil·i·ver·di·nate

bil·let

Bill·roth
    B's operation

bi·loph·odont

bi·max·il·lary

Bim·ler
    B. appliance
    B. stimulator

bin·an·gle

Bind·er
    B's syndrome

Bing
    B. bridge

Bio·blend ar·ti·fi·cial an·te·ri·or tooth molds

Bio·bond por·ce·lain

bio·com·pat·i·bil·i·ty

bio·film
    bacterial b.

Bio·form ex·tend·ed-range shade guide

bio·func·tion·al·i·ty

bio·glass

bio·in·te·gra·tion

bio·ma·te·ri·al

bio·me·chan·ics
    dental b.

Bio·mer ce·ment

bi·o·na·tor
    Balters b.

Bio-Oss

bio·phys·ics
    dental b.

bi·op·sy
    fine-needle aspiration b.

Bio-Vent im·plant

bi·phen·yl di·meth·ac·ry·late

bis·cuit
    hard b.
    high b.
    low b.
    medium b.
    soft b.

bis·cuit·ing

Bis·fil I com·pos·ite res·in

bis-GMA
    bisphenol-glycidyl
      methacrylate

Bish·op
    B. retractor

bisque
    high b.
    low b.
    medium b.

bis·muth

bite
    anterior deep b.
    anterior open b.
    balanced b.
    biscuit b.
    b. block
    check b.
    closed b.
    compound open b.
    convenience b.

bite *(continued)*
    cross b.
    deep b.
    dual b.
    edge-to-edge b.
    end-to-end b.
    b. guard
    infantile open b.
    lateral check b.
    locked b.
    mush b.
    open b.
    over b.
    raised b.
    raising b.
    rest b.
    b. rim
    scissors b.
    simple open b.
    skeletal deep b.
    skeletal open b.
    skeletal-type deep b.
    b. stick
    Sunday b.
    telescopic b.
    underhung b.
    wax b.
    X-b.

bite-block

bite-fork

bite·gage

bite·lock

bite·plane

bite·plate

bite-wing

bit·ing
    cheek b.
    lip b.
    b. pressure
    tongue b.

Bix·ler
    Antley-B. syndrome

Black
    B's formula (for identifying
       handcutting instruments)
    B. retractor
    B. wiring

blade
    carving b.
    endosteal implant b.
    b. implant
    knife b.
    scalpel b.

Blair
    B. incision
    B. knife

Bla·si·us
    B's duct

blas·to·my·co·sis

bleach·er

bleach·ing
    coronal b.

bleed·ing
    acute gingival b.
    chronic gingival b.
    gingival b.

BLEL
    benign lymphoepithelial
      lesion

Bliz·zard
    Johnson-B. syndrome

block
    autogenous bone b's
    autogenous
      corticocancellous bone b.
    bite b.
    corticocancellous onlay
      bone b's
    Gow-Gates mandibular b.
    greater palatine nerve b.

block·age
    apical b.

block·out
    arbitrary b.

block·out *(continued)*
    parallel b.
    shaped b.

Bloom
    B. syndrome

Blue Core Build Up Ma·te·ri·al

Blue Die Stone den·tal stone

Blue·phase-P

Blu·men·thal
    B. rongeur

Blu-Mousse im·pres·sion paste

BMP
    bone morphogenetic
      protein

board
    angle b.

Bock
    B's nerve

body
    adipose b. of cheek
    mandibular b.
    telobranchial b's

Bohn
    B's nodules

Boi·tel
    Steiger-B. attachment
    Steiger-B. bar

Bo·ley
    B. gauge
    modified B. gauge (MBG)

bolt
    denture b.
    P.W. (Pullen-Warner) b.

Bol·ton
    B. discrepancy
    B. point
    B. template
    B. triangle

bond
  Clearfil Porcelain B.

Bon·dent den·tin bond·ing pin

bond·ing
  direct b.
  indirect b.
  tooth b.

Bond·lite bond·ing sys·tem

bone
  AAA (autolyzed antigen-
    extracted allogeneic) b.
  alveolar b.
  autogenous
    corticocancellous b.
  basal b.
  bundle b.
  cancellous b.
  cortical b.
  demineralized b.
  demineralized freeze-dried
    b.
  ethmoid b.
  hyoid b.
  incisive b.
  jaw b., lower
  jaw b., upper
  Keil b.
  lamellar b.
  lamellated b.
  malar b.
  maxillary b.
  maxillary b., inferior
  maxillary b., superior
  palate b.
  palatine b.
  particulate b.
  premaxillary b.
  woven b.

Bon·will
  B. crown
  B. triangle

bo·plant

bor·der
  alveolar b. of mandible

bor·der (continued)
  alveolar b. of maxilla
  denture b.
  inferior b. of mandible
  b. molding

bo·ron
  b. carbide

Bos·ker TMI sys·tem

boss·ing

bou·gie
  Tucker b.

Bou·is·son
  B. apparatus

bow
  buccinator b.
  labial b.
  Logan b.

Bowles
  B. attachment
  B. bracket
  B. multiphase appliance
  B. multiphase attachment
  B. technique

Bow·man
  B's probe

Box
  B's technique

box·ing

Boyn·ton
  B. needle holder

BPDM
  biphenyl dimethacrylate

brace
  jab b.

brachy·ce·phal·ic

brachy·staph·y·line

brachy·uran·ic

brac·ing

brack·et
    Begg b.
    Bowles b.
    ceramic b.
    edgewise b.
    multiphase b.
    orthodontic b.
    ribbon arch b.
    twin-wire b.
    universal b.

Brack·ett
    B's probe

Bra·der
    B. arch form

branch
    alveolar b's of inferior
        alveolar artery
    anterior superior alveolar
        b's of infraorbital artery
    anterior superior alveolar
        b's of infraorbital nerve
    anterior superior dental b's
        of infraorbital nerve
    buccal b's of facial nerve
    dental b's of anterior
        superior alveolar arteries
    dental b's of inferior
        alveolar artery
    dental b's of posterior
        superior alveolar artery
    gingival b. of greater
        palatine artery
    gingival b. of posterior
        superior alveolar artery
    incisive b. of inferior
        alveolar nerve
    incisor b. of inferior
        alveolar artery
    inferior dental b's of
        inferior dental plexus
    inferior gingival b's of
        inferior dental plexus
    interdental b's
    interradicular b's
    middle superior alveolar b.
        of infraorbital nerve

branch (continued)
    middle superior dental b.
        of infraorbital nerve
    palatine b. of ascending
        pharyngeal artery
    perforating alveolar b's
    posterior superior alveolar
        b's of maxillary nerve
    posterior superior dental
        b's of maxillary nerve
    superior dental b's of
        superior dental plexus
    superior gingival b's of
        superior dental plexus

bran·chi·al

Bråne·mark
    B. implants
    B. Implant System

Bra·zil wax

breadth
    anterior b. of mandible
    bicanine b.
    bigonial b.
    bimolar b.
    bizygomatic b.
    condylar b. of mandible
    cranial b.
    b. of mandible
    b. of mandibular ramus
    maxilloalveolar b.
    midfacial b.
    b. of palate
    zygomatic b.

break·er
    stress b.

B-1 ream·er

B-2 ream·er

breath
    bad b.

breath·ing
    mouth b.

Bre·vais
    B. lattice

Bre·vi·tal

Brew·er
    B's forceps

bridge
    Aderer 'C' B.
    American Gold "B" B.
    American Gold "T" B.
        Hard
    Andrews b.
    Bing b.
    cantilever b.
    complex b.
    compound b.
    cross b.
    dental b.
    dentin b.
    extension b.
    fixed b.
    fixed-fixed b.
    fixed-movable b.
    fixed b. with rigid
        connectors
    fixed b. with rigid and
        nonrigid connectors
    hydrogen b.
    intercellular b.
    Libra III Crown and B.
    b. of the nose
    removable b.
    spring b.
    stationary b.

Bridge III-C gold al·loy

Bridge Par·tial IV-D gold al·
    loy

bridge·work
    fixed b.
    removable b.

bridg·ing
    dentinal b.

Brin·ell
    B. hardness indenter point
    B. hardness number
        (BHN)
    B. hardness scale

Brin·ell (continued)
    B. hardness test
    B. indenter
    B. indenter point
    B. scale

Brink·er tis·sue re·trac·tors

bris·tle
    hard b.
    natural b.
    nylon b.
    soft b.

broach
    barbed b.
    Dry Guard Virilium Union
        B.
    endodontic b.
    pathfinder b.
    root canal b.
    smooth b.

Broad·bent
    B. registration point

Bro·ca
    B's point

Bro·ders
    B. classification (for
        malignancy)

Bro·dy
    B's syndrome

brom·op·nea

Brook air·way-re·sus·ci·tat·
    ing tube

Bro·phy
    B's operation

Brosch
    B. procedure

Brown
    Adson-B. forceps

Brown·ie den·tal stone

brow·pexy

brush
    Bass' b.
    Benda B.
    bristle b.
    b. condensation
    denture b.
    interproximal b.
    polishing b.
    tooth b.
    wire b.

brush·ing

brush-on

brux

brux·ism
    centric b.
    eccentric b.

bruxo·ma·nia

BSSO
    bilateral sagittal split
    osteotomy

buc·cal

buc·cal·ly

buc·co·ax·i·al

buc·co·ax·io·cer·vi·cal

buc·co·ax·io·gin·gi·val

buc·co·cer·vi·cal

buc·co·clu·sal

buc·co·clu·sion

buc·co·dis·tal

buc·co·gin·gi·val

buc·co·la·bi·al

buc·co·lin·gual

buc·co·lin·gual·ly

buc·co·max·il·lary

buc·co·me·si·al

buc·co-oc·clu·sal

buc·co·phar·yn·ge·al

buc·co·place·ment

buc·co·pul·pal

buc·co·ver·sion

Buck
    B. knife
    B. wiring

Buck·ley type for·mo·cre·sol

bu·lim·ia

bul·lous

bump·er
    lip b.

BUN
    blood urea nitrogen

bun·dle
    alveolar neurovascular b.

Bung·ner
    bands of B.

bu·piv·a·caine

bur
    ACORDE b.
    all purpose b.
    amalgam prep b.
    barrel b.
    bone b.
    bud b.
    bullet b.
    carbide b.
    cone course b.
    cone shape b.
    crosscut b.
    crosscut fissure b.
    crosscut straight fissure b.
    crosscut taper fissure b.
    crosscut tapered fissure b.
    cylinder b.
    dentate b.
    dentate straight fissure b.
    dentate tapered fissure b.
    diamond b.
    egg b.
    end-cutting fissure b.
    endodontic b.

bur *(continued)*
    excavating b.
    extra long taper b.
    Feldman b.
    fine finishing b.
    fine finishing ball b.
    fine finishing needle long
      b.
    fine finishing straight
      dome b.
    finishing b.
    fissure b.
    flame b.
    flat end fissure b.
    Gates Glidden b.
    Goldies carbide b.
    inlay prep b.
    inverted cone b.
    inverted pear b.
    inverted taper b.
    lab b.
    Lindemann b.
    Magician b.
    needle b.
    oval b.
    pear b.
    pear-shaped b.
    plain fissure b.
    plain round b.
    plain straight fissure b.
    plain tapered fissure b.
    plain taper fissure b.
    plug-finishing b.
    pointed cone b.
    resin b.
    restoration removal b.
    round end fissure b.
    round taper b.
    Starlite Omni-AT b.
    straight dome b.
    straight dome crosscut b.
    straight finishing b.
    straight fissure b.
    surgical b.
    taper b.
    taper dome b.
    taper finishing b.

bur *(continued)*
    taper fissure b.
    taper fissure crosscut b.
    trimming and finishing b.

Bu·reau of Health In·sur·ance

Bu·reau of Qual·i·ty As·sur·
ance

Bur·kitt
    B's cell acute leukemia
    B's lymphoma

Bur·lew disk

Bur·lew wheel

Bur·ling·ton
    B. growth study

burn
    aspirin b's
    chemical b.
    egg shape b.
    electrical b.
    end cutting b.

Bur·nett
    B. ratchet device

bur·nish·er
    agate b.
    amalgam b.
    fishtail b.
    fissure b.
    flat b.
    gold b.
    straight b.

bur·nish·ing

burn·out
    wax b.

Burns Uni·file

burr

bur·sa *pl.* bur·sae
    Fleischmann's b.

Bur·stone
    B's arch technique
    Legan and B.
      cephalometric standards

but·ton
   lingual b.
   palatal b.

but·tress
   zygomatic b.

but·tress·ing
   b. bone formation

BW gauge

Byz·an·tine pal·ate

CAD/CAM
  computer-aided design/
    computer-aided
    manufacturing

Caf·fey
  C. syndrome

cal·ci·fi·ca·tion
  pulp c.

Cal·cio·bi·ot·ic root ca·nal seal·er

Cal·ci·tite

cal·ci·um
  c. chloride
  c. hydroxide
  c. pyrophosphate
  c. pyrophosphate dihydrate
  c. triphosphate

cal·cu·lus
  dental c.

Cald·well
  C.-Luc operation

cal·i·per
  Beerendonk c.
  Vernier c.

Cal·la·han
  C. method
  Johnston-C. diffusion
    technique

cam·era *pl.* **cam·eras, cam· erae**
  Dentacam I intraoral c.
  Dentacam II intraoral c.
  intraoral c.

Ca·na·di·an Den·tal As·so·ci· a·tion

ca·nal
  accessory palatine c's
  accessory root c.

ca·nal *(continued)*
  alveolar c's
  alveolar c., anterior
  alveolar c. of maxilla
  bayonet c.
  bayonet root c.
  branching c.
  C-shaped c.
  C-shaped root c.
  curved c.
  curved root c.
  dental c., inferior
  dental c's, posterior
  dentinal c's
  dilacerated c.
  dilacerated root c.
  gubernacular c's
  haversian c.
  Hirschfeld's c's
  interdental c's
  mandibular c.
  nasolacrimal c.
  pulp c.
  radicular c.
  c's of Rivinus
  root c.
  root c. disinfection
  root c. sterilization
  root c. therapy
  secondary c.
  sickle-shaped c.

Can-a-Seal ce·ment

can·cer
  oral c.

Can·di·da
  C. albicans
  C. stellatoides
  C. tropicalis

can·di·di·a·sis
  oral c.

can·di·do·sis
  pseudomembranous c.

ca·nine

ca·ni·nus

cant
  c. of mandible

can·thot·o·my

cap
  enamel c.
  germinal c.
  c. splint

ca·pit·u·lum *pl.* ca·pit·u·la
  c. [processus condyloidei]
    mandibulae

Cap·mix mix·ing unit

cap·ping
  direct pulp c.
  indirect pulp c.
  pulp c.

cap·su·la *pl.* cap·su·lae
  c. articularis mandibulae

cap·ut *pl.* cap·i·ta
  c. angulare musculi
    quadrati labii superioris
  c. infraorbitale musculi
    quadrati labii superioris
  c. progeneum
  c. zygomaticum musculi
    quadrati labii superioris

Ca·ra·bel·li
  C. cusp
  C's sign
  C. tubercle

car·ba·maz·e·pine

car·ba·mide
  c. peroxide

Car·ba·pen·ems

car·ben·i·cil·lin

Car·bide Ste·ri·bur

Car·bo·caine

car·bon
  vitreous c.

car·bo·pla·tin

Car·bo·run·dum disk

car·ci·no·ma *pl.* car·ci·no·mas,
  car·ci·no·ma·ta
  acinar cell c.
  acinic cell c.
  acinous cell c.
  adenocystic basal cell c.
  adenoid cystic c.
  ameloblastic c.
  c. arising in odontogenic
    cysts
  basal cell c.
  basaloid salivary c.
  central adenoid cystic c.
  epidermoid c.
  c. ex mixed tumor
  c. in situ
  intraosseous
    mucoepidermoid c.
  lobular c.
  mucoepidermoid c.
  nasopharyngeal c.
  oral squamous cell c's
    (OSCC)
  primary intraosseous c.
  pseudoadenomatous basal
    cell c.
  sinus c.
  spindle cell c.
  squamous cell c.
  terminal duct c.
  verrucous c.

care
  adequate dental c.
  comprehensive dental c.
  dental c.
  emergency dental c.
  incremental dental c.
  initial dental c.
  maintenance dental c.
  minimal dental c.
  primary dental c.

car·ies
  pit c.
  radiation c.

Car·pen·ter
  C. syndrome

car·ri·er
  amalgam c.
  foil c.
  lentulo paste c.
  paste c.
  Syncote amalgam c.

Car·roll
  C.-Girard screw

Car·ter
  C's intranasal splint

car·ti·lage
  alar c.
  articular c.
  arytenoid c.
  cricoid c.
  dentinal c.
  gingival c.

ca·run·cu·la *pl.* ca·run·cu·lae
  c. salivaris

car·ver
  amalgam c.
  anatomical c.
  cleoid c.
  discoid c.
  IPC interproximal c.
  knife-bladed c.
  Martin c.
  Roach c.
  ruby c.
  TC (tungsten carbide) c.
  TC-A c.
  TC-B c.
  TC-C c.
  TC-D c.
  TC-E c.
  Vehe c.
  wax c.

carv·ing

Case
  C's enamel cleaver
  C's velum obturator

case

Cas·pers·son
  C. technique

cas·sette

cast
  dental c.
  diagnostic c.
  gnathostatic c.
  implant c.
  c. investment
  investment c.
  master c.
  modified c.
  preextraction c.
  preoperative c.
  refractory c.
  study c.
  study implant c.
  working c.

cast·ing
  gold alloy dental c.
  c. machine
  c. ring
  superstructure c.
  vacuum c.

Cast·mat·ic-S ti·ta·ni·um cast·ing sys·tem

Cas·tro·vie·jo
  C. needle holder

cat·a·lyst
  dual-cure c.

Cat·to·ni
  C. scaler

Caul·field
  C. retriever

Caulk im·pres·sion paste

Caulk Mi·cro II

Caulk Op·ta·loy

Caulk Op·ta·loy II

Caulk spher·i·cal al·loy

Caulk Syn·trex F

Caulk var·nish

cau·tery
    McCain bipolar c.

Cav·a·lite cav·i·ty lin·er

cave
    Meckel's c.

cav·er·nous

Ca·vi·dry

Cavi-Jet

cav·i·tas *pl.* cav·i·ta·tes
    c. oris externa

Cav·it ce·ment

Ca·vi·tec cav·i·ty lin·er

Cav·it fill·ing ma·te·ri·al

Cav·it G ce·ment

Cav·it G tem·po·rary fill·ing
    ma·te·ri·al

Ca·vi-Trol acid·u·lat·ed phos·
    phate flu·o·ride top·i·cal gel

Cav·i·tron unit

Cav·it tem·po·rary fill·ing ma·
    te·ri·al

Cav·it W ce·ment

Cav·it W tem·po·rary fill·ing
    ma·te·ri·al

cav·i·ty
    access c.
    alveolar c's
    axial surface c.
    buccal c.
    c. classification
    complex c.
    compound c.
    c. débridement

cav·i·ty *(continued)*
    dental c.
    distal c.
    DO (disto-occlusal) c.
    endodontic c.
    faucial c.
    fissure c.
    gingival c.
    gingival third c.
    incisal c.
    infraglottic c.
    labial c.
    lingual c.
    c. lining agent
    mesial c.
    MO (mesio-occlusal) c.
    MOD (mesio-occlusodistal)
        c.
    nerve c.
    NICO c's
    occlusal c.
    oral c.
    oral c., external
    pit c.
    prepared c.
    c. primer
    proximal c.
    pulp c.
    c. seal
    simple c.
    smooth surface c.

ca·vum *pl.* ca·va
    c. oris externum

CBA No. 9080 ce·ment

C&B Meta·bond ad·he·sive
    res·in

CDA
    Certified Dental Assistant

CDT
    Certified Dental
        Technician

cef·o·tax·ime

Ce·ka at·tach·ment

Ce·ka Bond

cell
- cement c.
- dentin c.
- giant c.
- Langerhans c's
- plasma c's
- Schwann c.
- xanthoma c.

cel·lu·li·tis
- facial and cervical c.

cel·lu·lose
- oxidized regenerated c.

cel·lu·los·ic acid

Cel·lu·meth

ce·ment
- ASPA c.
- Biomer c.
- black copper c.
- calcium hydroxide c.
- Can-a-Seal c.
- Cavit c.
- Cavit G c.
- Cavit W c.
- CBA No. 9080 c.
- C&B Metabond adhesive c.
- Cimpat c.
- Comspan composite luting c.
- Comspan luting c.
- dental c.
- dimethacrylate c.
- Durelon c.
- Durelon carboxylate c.
- EBA c.
- Elite c.
- EMKA-Base glass ionomer c.
- EMKA-Silver glass ionomer c.
- endodontic c.
- Flecks c.
- Flexi-Flow c.
- Flexi-Flow composite c.
- Flow-Temp c.
- Fluoro-Thin c.

ce·ment *(continued)*
- fortified zinc oxide-eugenol c.
- Fuji I luting c.
- Fuji lining glass ionomer c.
- Fuji lining LC c.
- Fynal c.
- GlasIonomer c.
- glass ionomer c.
- glass ionomer luting c.
- Grip c.
- Hy-Bond c.
- Hy-Bond polycarboxylate c.
- Hy-Bond zinc oxide eugenol temporary c.
- Hy-Bond zinc phosphate c.
- hydrophosphate c.
- improved zinc oxide–eugenol c.
- Insure resin c.
- Interval c.
- Ionoscem c.
- Justi Resin c.
- Kent zinc c.
- Ketac-Bond c.
- Ketac-Bond Aplicap c.
- Ketac-Cem Aplicap c.
- Ketac-Cem MAXICAP c.
- Ketac-Cem radiopaque c.
- lining c.
- modified zinc oxide–eugenol c.
- modified zinc phosphate c.
- MQ c.
- Mynol c.
- Neo-Temp c.
- NOgenol c.
- Panavia luting c.
- PMMA (polymethyl methacrylate) c.
- polycarboxylate c.
- polymethyl methacrylate c.
- porcelain c.
- Porcelite c.
- Proviscell c.
- pseudocopper c.
- red copper c.

ce·ment *(continued)*
    reinforced zinc oxide-
      eugenol c.
    Resiment c.
    resin c.
    root canal c.
    silicate c.
    silicate zinc c.
    silicophosphate c.
    Smith's resin c.
    Smith's zinc c.
    Temp-Bond c.
    Temp-Bond NE c.
    Tempak c.
    Temrex c.
    Tenacin c.
    Tylok-Plus c.
    U/P root canal c.
    zinc c.
    zinc oxide–eugenol c.
    zinc phosphate c.
    zinc polyacrylate c.
    zinc polycarboxylate c.
    zinc silicophosphate c.
    ZOE (zinc oxide–eugenol)
      c.
    ZOE type temporary c.

ce·men·tal

ce·men·ta·tion

ce·men·ti·cle
    adherent c.
    attached c.
    free c.
    interstitial c.

ce·men·ti·fi·ca·tion

ce·men·ti·tis

ce·men·to·blast

ce·men·to·blas·to·ma

ce·men·to·cla·sia

ce·men·to·clast

ce·men·to·cyte

ce·men·to·gen·e·sis

ce·men·toid

ce·men·to·ma
    gigantiform c.
    gigantiform monstrous c.
    true c.

ce·men·to·path·ia

ce·men·to·peri·os·ti·tis

ce·men·to·sis

ce·men·tum
    aberrant c.
    acellular c.
    afibrillar c.
    cellular c.
    coronal c.
    intermediate c.
    primary c.
    root c.
    secondary c.
    uncalcified c.

cen·ter
    dentary c.
    facial c.
    freedom in c.

cen·tric
    acquired c.
    broad c.
    habitual c.
    long c.
    Myo-Monitor c.
    c. occlusion
    c. position
    power c.
    c. relation
    retruded c.
    slide in c.
    true c.

CEOT
    calcifying epithelial
      odontogenic tumor

ceph·a·lex·in

ceph·a·lo·gram
    lateral c.

ce·pha·log·ra·phy

ceph·a·lom·e·ter

ceph·a·lo·met·ric

ce·pha·lo·met·rics

ceph·a·lom·e·try
    craniofacial c.

ceph·a·lo·spo·rin
    c. C
    c. N
    c. P

ceph·a·lo·stat

Ce·ram·co body shades

Ce·ram·co II por·ce·lain

ce·ram·ic
    dental c.
    glass c.
    P-50 light cured resin
        bonded c.

ce·ram·ics
    calcium phosphate c.
    dental c.
    hydroxyapatite c.

Ce·ram·isté cup

Ce·ram·isté point

Ce·ram·isté wheel

ce·ram·odon·tics

ce·ramo·me·tal

Ce·rec CAD/CAM sys·tem

ce·res·in

Cer·ti·fy·ing Board of the
    Amer·i·can Den·tal As·sis·
    tants As·so·ci·a·tion

cer·vi·co·buc·cal

cer·vi·co·la·bi·al

cer·vi·co·lin·gual

Cer·vi·dent bond·ing sys·tem

Ce·ta·caine

ce·tyl-di·meth·yl·ben·zyl-am·
    mo·ni·um chlo·ride

C-form os·te·ot·o·my

chair
    dental c.

chair·side

chalk
    French c.
    precipitated c.

cham·ber
    bone growth c.
    pulp c.
    relief c.

cham·fer

Cham·py
    C. plates

Chan·dler
    C. chisel

CHARGE as·so·ci·a·tion

chart
    dental c.
    periodontal c.

Char·ters
    C. method of
        toothbrushing
    C. technique

Chayes
    C. attachment

check-bite

Check-Bite tray

chei·lec·to·my

chei·li·tis
    angular c.
    exfoliative c.
    c. glandularis
    c. granulomatosa

chei·lo·plas·ty

chei·lo·rhi·no·plas·ty

chei·lor·rha·phy

chei·lo·sis
    actinic c.

chei·lo·sto·ma·to·plas·ty

chei·lot·o·my

Che·lon-Sil·ver

Chem·i·clave

Che·ney
    Hajdu-C. syndrome

cher·ub·ism

CHILD syn·drome

chin·cap

chip
    bone c's
    cortical c's

chis·el
    binangle c.
    binangled c.
    bone c.
    Chandler c.
    contra-angle c.
    curved c.
    Kirkland c.
    monangle c.
    Ochsenbein c.
    periodontal c.
    Rhodes back action c.
    Sorensen c.
    straight c.
    TG/O c.
    Wedelstaedt c.

chi·to·san

chlo·ral hy·drate

chlor·hex·i·dine
    c. gluconate

chlo·ri·dia·ze·pox·ide

chlo·ro·bu·ta·nol

Chlo·ro·form

chlo·ro·ma

chlo·ro·per·cha

p-chlo·ro·phe·nol [para-]
    camphorated p-c.

chlo·ro·quine

Chlo·ro-Thy·mo·nol root ca·nal
    dress·ing

chlor·tet·ra·cy·cline

cho·le·ste·a·to·ma

cho·line
    c. salicylate

chon·dro·cra·ni·um

chon·dro·dys·pla·sia
    metaphyseal c., Jansen
        type
    c. punctata

chon·dro·ma

chon·dro·ma·to·sis
    synovial c.

chon·dro·ma·tous

chon·dro·meta·pla·sia

chon·dro·myx·o·ma

chon·dro·sar·co·ma
    mesenchymal c.

chord
    condyle c.

cho·ris·to·ma
    chondromatous c.
    osseous c.

Chot·zen
    Saethre-C. syndrome

Chris·ten·sen
    C. articulator

Chris·tian
    Hand-Schüller-C. disease

chrome
    cobalt c.

chro·mi·um

Chvos·tek
    C. sign

Cim·pat ce·ment

Cinch-Vi·nyl im·pres·sion ma·
    te·ri·al

Cinch-Vi·nyl vi·nyl poly·
    siloxane im·pres·sion ma·te·
    ri·al paste

cin·gu·la

cin·gu·lum *pl.*cin·gu·la
    c. dentis

cin·na·mon

Cip·ro

cip·ro·flox·a·cin

cir·cle
    centigrade c.

CI-S
    simplified calculus index

Ci·ta·nest

Ci·ta·nest For·te

Cit·ri·con im·pres·sion ma·te·
    ri·al

Cla·fo·ran

clamp
    cervical c.
    cotton roll rubber dam c.
    Crile's c.
    Ferrier 212 gingival c.
    gingival c.
    Hatch c.
    Ivory c.
    Joseph's c.
    pedicle c.
    root rubber dam c.
    rubber dam c.
    S.S.W. c.
    S.S. White c.

Clark
    C. attachment
    C's rule

clasp
    Adams c.
    Aderer No. 20 c.
    arrow c.
    arrowhead c.
    back-action c.
    ball c.
    bar c.
    cast c.
    circumferential c.
    combination c.
    continuous c.
    continuous lingual c.
    Crozat c.
    embrassure c.
    formed c.
    c. guideline
    hairpin c.
    half-and-half c.
    infrabulge c.
    mesiodistal c.
    movable c.
    movable-arm c.
    multiple c.
    c. No. 4
    c. No. 18
    retentive c.
    reverse-action c.
    ring c.
    Roach c.
    wrought c.

Clasp Wire

clas·si·fi·ca·tion
    Ackerman-Proffit c. (for
        malocclusion)
    American Cleft Palate
        Association c.
    Angle's c. (for
        malocclusion)
    Bailyn's c. (for partially
        edentulous arches)
    Broders' c. (for
        malignancy)
    cleft palate c.
    Kennedy c. (for partially
        edentulous arches)
    salivary tumor c.

clas·si·fi·ca·tion *(continued)*
    Schwarz's c. (of orthodontic
      forces)
    Skinner's c. (for partially
      edentulous arches)
    c. of soft tissue tumors
    Stark c. (for cleft palate)
    Veau c. (for cleft palate)

Class I stone

Class II stone

C & L at·tach·ment

cla·vu·lan·ate
    c. potassium

cleans·er
    abrasive denture c.
    alkaline hypochlorite
      denture c.
    alkaline peroxide denture
      c.
    denture c.
    dilute acid denture c.
    immersion denture c.
    Proxigel oral antiseptic c.
    ultrasonic denture c.

cleans·ing
    occlusal c.

clear·ance
    interocclusal c.
    occlusal c.

Clear·fil Pho·to-Bond bond·ing
  sys·tem

Clear·fil Por·ce·lain Bond

cleat

cleav·er
    Case's enamel c.
    Orton's enamel c.

cleft
    alveolar c.
    bilateral c.
    facial c's
    gingival c.
    interdental c.

cleft *(continued)*
    lateral facial c.
    midline maxillary c.
    oblique facial c.
    postalveolar c.
    prealveolar c.
    Stillman's c.

clei·do·cra·ni·al

clench·ing
    habitual c.

cle·oid

click
    eminence c.
    temporomandibular joint c.

click·ing

clin·da·my·cin

clo·ni·dine hy·dro·chlo·ride

clos·trid·i·um *pl.* clos·trid·ia

clo·sure
    flask c.
    flask c., final
    flask c., trial
    palatal c.
    V-Y c.
    Y-c.

cloth
    squeeze c.

clo·trim·a·zole

C & L unit

clus·ter

C & M 637 at·tach·ment

CM en·dos·se·ous im·plant

CM im·plant

CML
    chronic myelogenous
      leukemia

coating
    Air Barrier C. (ABC)

co·balt
  c. chrome

co·caine

coc·cid·i·oi·do·my·co·sis

Cock·ayne
  C's syndrome

code
  ADA Uniform C. on Dental
    Procedures and
    Nomenclature

Coe al·gi·nate

Coe bite reg·is·tra·tion creme

Coe·cal den·tal stone

Coe Com·fort den·ture re·lin·
  er

Coe Com·fort eden·tu·lous tis·
  sue con·di·tion·er

Coe Cure re·pair res·in

Coe-flex im·pres·sion ma·te·ri·
  al

Coe Flo im·pres·sion paste

Coe hy·dro·phil·ic gel

Coe Or·tho res·in

Coe-Pak Au·to·mix peri·odon·
  tal dress·ing

Coe-Pak paste

Coe Rect den·ture lin·er

Coe-soft den·ture lin·er

Coe-soft den·ture re·lin·er

Cof·fin
  C. appliance
  C. plate
  C. split plate
  C. spring
  C.-Lowry syndrome
  C.-Siris syndrome

Co·hen
  C. syndrome

col

Col·burn
  Miller-C. file

co·li·tis pl. co·lit·i·des
  ulcerative c.

Col·la·Cote col·la·gen wound
  dress·ing

col·la·gen

Col·la·Plug col·la·gen wound
  dress·ing

Col·la·Tape col·la·gen wound
  dress·ing

Col·la-Tec ab·sorb·able col·la·
  gen dress·ing

Col·lier
  C. needle holder

col·loid

col·lum pl. col·la
  c. dentis
  c. processus condyloidei
    mandibulae

col·or
  tooth c.

Co·lum·bia cu·ret

Co·lum·bia re·trac·tor

col·umn
  enamel c's

Com·man·do
  C's operation

com·mis·sion
  c's of the American Dental
    Association

Com·mis·sion on Den·tal Ac·
  cred·i·ta·tion of the Amer·i·
  can Den·tal As·so·ci·a·tion

com·mit·tee
  dental review c.

com·pact

com·pac·tion
  direct filling gold c.

com·par·a·tor
  Dental Shade C.

com·plex
  inclusion c's
  maxillo-craniofacial c.
  zygomatic c.

com·po·nent
  anterior c.

Com·po·shape fin·ish·ing sys·tem

com·pos·ite
  Concise c.
  Degufil H c.
  Degufil M c.
  Fermit c.
  Geristone C.
  Herculite XR c.
  Herculite XRV c.
  P-10 c.
  P-10 resin bonded ceramic
    c.
  Prisma AP.H c.

com·pound
  block out c.
  impression c.
  modeling c.
  tray c.
  true impression c.
  c. Type I
  c. Type II

com·pres·sion

Com·span com·pos·ite lut·ing
  ce·ment

Com·span lut·ing ce·ment

Con·cise com·pos·ite

Con·cise crown build-up

Con·cise light cured white seal·ant

Con·cise or·tho·don·tic bond·ing sys·tem

Con·cise seal·ant

Con·cise white seal·ant res·in

Con·cise white seal·ant sys·tem

con·cres·cence

con·den·sa·tion
  brush c.
  filling material c.
  gold foil c.
  hand amalgam c.
  mechanical amalgam c.
  c. polymerization
  porcelain c.
  pressure c.
  c. resin
  spatulation c.
  vibration c.
  whipping c.

con·den·ser
  amalgam c.
  automatic c.
  back-action c.
  bayonet c.
  electromallet c.
  foot c.
  gold c.
  hand c.
  Hollenback c.
  mechanical c.
  mechanical gold c.
  parallelogram c.
  pneumatic c.
  c. point
  reverse c.
  root canal filling c.
  round c.

con·di·tion·er
  Barrier dentin c.
  Coe Comfort edentulous
    tissue c.

con·di·tion·er *(continued)*
Getz dentin c.
Lynal tissue c.
Nuva-System Tooth c.
Recon tissue c. and functional impression material
Softone tissue c. and functional impression material
Visco-gel tissue c. and liner

con·dy·lar

con·dyle
double c.
c. of mandible
mandibular c.

con·dy·lec·to·my

con·dyl·i·on

con·dy·lo·ma *pl.* con·dy·lo·ma·ta
c. acuminatum
c. latum

con·dy·lot·o·my

cone
compound c.
cutting c.
felt c.
gutta-percha c.
long c.
short c.
silver c's

Co·nex at·tach·ment

con·flu·ence
apical c.

con·gen·i·ta

con·gen·i·tal

con·nec·tor
anterior major palatal c.
arch bar splint c.
c. bar
double major c.

con·nec·tor *(continued)*
implant superstructure c.
major c.
major palatal c.
minor c.
nonrigid c.
palatal c.
posterior major palatal c.
rigid c.
saddle c.
split major c.
Steiger's c.
subocclusal c.
superstructure c.

con·stric·tion
transverse maxillary c.

con·stric·ture
apical c.

con·struc·tion
skeletal maxillary c.

con·tact
c. area
balancing c.
complete c.
deflective c.
deflective occlusal c.
direct c.
faulty c.
faulty interproximal c.
immediate direct c.
initial c.
initial occlusal c.
interceptive occlusal c.
interproximal c.
mediate c.
occlusal c.
c. point
occlusal c., deflective
occlusal c., initial
occlusal c., interceptive
premature c.
proximal c.
proximate c.
weak c.
working c.

con·tour
  buccal c.
  chin c.
  facial c.
  gingival c.
  gingival denture c.
  height of c.
  proximal c.

Con·tour al·loy

con·tour·ing
  occlusal c.

con·tra-an·gle

con·trac·tion

Cook-Waite as·pi·rat·ing sy·ringe

cool·ant
  tooth c.

COP
  chronic obstructive
    parotitis

co·pal

Co·pal cav·i·ty var·nish

Co·pa·lite var·nish

cope

cop·ing
  paralleling c.
  primary c.
  telescopic c.
  transfer c's

Copr·wax bite wa·fer

Cora-Caine

cord
  Gingipak retraction c.
  Pascord retraction c.
  Racord retraction c.
  retraction c.
  Retrax retraction c.
  Retreat II retraction cord
  Retreat retraction c.
  Sil-Trax retraction c.

cord *(continued)*
  Sulpak retraction c.
  WEDJETS dental dam c.

core
  cast c.
  disappearing c.
  pulp c.

Core-Vent im·plant

co·ro·ne

co·ro·ni·on

cor·o·noid

cor·o·noi·dec·to·my

cor·o·noi·dot·o·my

cor·po·ra·tion
  dental service c.

cor·rec·tion
  occlusal c.

cor·rec·tor
  function c.

Cor·ri·gan
  C's line

cor·ti·cal·os·te·ot·o·my

cor·ti·cot·o·my
  midpalatal c.

co·run·dum

Cos·mic Bond bond·ing sys·tem

Cos·ten
  C's syndrome

coun·ter·die

cou·ple

coup·ler
  silane c.

cov·er·age
  denture c.
  occlusal c.

Cow·den
  C's syndrome

CPPD
  calcium pyrophosphate
    dihydrate

CR
  centric relation

Crane
  C. pick elevator
  C. Kaplan scaler

cra·nio·fa·cial

cra·nio·man·dib·u·lar

Cra·nio·plast

cra·nio·syn·os·to·sis
  unilateral lambdoid c.

cra·ter
  alveolar process c.
  bone c.
  gingival c.
  interalveolar bone c.

craz·ing
  resin c.

CRCS
  calciobiotic root canal
    sealer

crease
  preauricular skin c.

cre·at·i·nine

creep
  dynamic c.
  static c.

cre·o·sote
  Beechwood c.

crep·i·ta·tion

Cre·sa·nol root ca·nal dress·
  ing

cre·sa·tin

cres·cent
  sublingual c.

crest
  alveolar c.
  buccinator c.
  gingival c.
  mental c., external

CREST syn·drome

m-cre·syl ace·tate

crev·ice
  gingival c.

cre·vic·u·lar

crib
  allogeneic bone c's
  allogeneic c.
  allogeneic mandible c's
  alloplastic c's
  Jackson c.
  lip-sucking habit c.
  metallic c's
  tongue c.

cri·co·thy·roi·dot·o·my

Crile
  C. clamp
  C. hemostat
  C.-Wood needle holder

Cris·ma·ni
  C. attachment
  C. combined attachment
  C. combined unit
  C. stress-breaker

cris·ta *pl.* cris·tae
  c. buccinatoria

CRMI
  centric relation maximum
    intercuspation

Crohn
  C's disease

Cross
  C. syndrome

cross·bite
  anterior c.
  buccal c.

cross·bite *(continued)*
  lingual c.
  posterior c.
  scissors-bite c.
  telescoping c.
  unilateral c.

Crou·zon
  C. syndrome

crowd·ing

crown
  anatomical c.
  artificial c.
  basket c.
  bell c.
  Bonwill c.
  cap c.
  celluloid c.
  clinical c.
  collar c.
  complete c.
  complete veneer c.
  Davis c.
  dental c.
  dowel c.
  extra-alveolar c.
  c. flask
  full c.
  full veneer c.
  gold shell c.
  half c.
  half-cap c.
  jacket c.
  c. length
  Libra II inlay and c.
  Libra III c. and bridge
  metal-ceramic c.
  open-face c.
  overlay c.
  partial c.
  partial veneer c.
  physiological c.
  pinledge c.
  porcelain-faced c.
  porcelain-faced dowel c.
  porcelain-fused-to-metal
    (PFM) c.

crown *(continued)*
  porcelain veneer gold c.
  post c.
  Richmond c.
  shell c.
  shoulderless jacket c.
  steel c.
  tapered c.
  telescopic c.
  temporary c.
  temporary acrylic c.
  thimble c.
  three-quarter c.
  veneer c., complete
  veneer c., full
  veneer c., partial
  veneered c.
  veneer metal c.
  Weston c.
  window c.

Crown amal·ga·ma·tor

Crown No. 1 gold al·loy

Crown No. 3 gold al·loy

Crown Hy·las·tic gold al·loy

Crown K in·lay

Crown Knapp No. 3 gold al·loy

Crown Su·preme gold al·loy

Crown TT gold al·loy

Cro·zat
  C. appliance
  C. clasp

cro·zat

Cry·er
  C. elevator
  C. forceps

crypt
  bony c.
  dental c.
  enamel c.
  tooth c.

cryp·to·coc·co·sis
  oral c.

C-shaped ca·nal

C-shaped root ca·nal

CSP
  channel shoulder pin
  crown shoulder pin

CSP at·tach·ment

CSP tech·nique

cu·cur·bi·tol

cuff
  attached epithelial c.
  attached gingival c.
  epithelial c.
  gingival c.
  gum c.

cup
  Ceramisté c.
  chin c.

Cu·pral·loy

cure

cu·ret
  Barnhart c.
  Columbia c.
  Goldman-Fox c.
  Gracey c's
  Implacare c.
  Kirkland c.
  Lucas c.
  McCall c.
  Miller c.
  Molt c.
  periodontal c.
  Prichard c.
  root planing c.
  scaling c.
  surgical c.
  universal c.
  Younger-Goode c.

Cure-Thru Wedge Sys·tem

cu·ret·tage
  apical c.
  gingival c.
  periapical c.
  soft tissue c.
  subgingival c.
  surgical c.
  ultrasonic c.

cu·rette

cur·ing
  denture c.
  visible light c.

cur·va·ture
  compensating c.
  occlusal c.

curve
  alignment c.
  anti-Monson c.
  apical c.
  bayonet c.
  buccal c.
  compensating c.
  defalcated c.
  dental c.
  dilacerated c.
  double c.
  dromedary c.
  elastic c.
  forced deflection c.
  gradual c.
  labial c.
  liquidus c.
  milled-in c.
  Monson c.
  c. of occlusion
  Pleasure c.
  reverse c.
  reverse c. of Spee
  sickle-shaped c.
  solidus c.
  c. of Spee
  stress-strain c.
  tension c's
  c. of Wilson

Cush·ing
   C's disease
   C. elevator

cush·ion
   sucking c.

Cu-Sil at·tach·ment

cusp
   accessory buccal c.
   Carabelli c.
   centric c's
   dental c.
   interstitial c.
   noncentric c's
   nonsupporting c's
   c. plane
   plunger c.
   shoeing c.
   supporting c's
   talon c.
   tipping c.

cus·pid

cus·pi·date

cus·pi·des

cus·pi·dor

cus·pis *pl.* cus·pi·des
   c. coronae
   c. dentis

cu·ti·cle
   dental c.
   enamel c.
   primary c.
   c. of root sheath
   secondary c.

cut·ter
   pin and ligature c.

Cut·ter·Jel al·gi·nate

Cut·ter·Jel im·pres·sion ma·te·ri·al

Cut·ter·Sil im·pres·sion ma·te·ri·al

Cut·ter·Sil Mu·co·sa im·pres·sion ma·te·ri·al

Cut·ter·Sil Mu·co·sa sil·i·cone im·pres·sion ma·te·ri·al

Cut·ter·Sil Put·ty

Cut·ter·Sil Put·ty Plus

Cut·ter·Sil XL im·pres·sion ma·te·ri·al

Cut·ter·Sil XL sil·i·cone im·pres·sion ma·te·ri·al

Cy·a·no·dent

cy·cle
   chewing c.
   masticating c.
   masticatory c.

cy·clo·phos·pha·mide

cy·clo·spo·rine

cy·no·dont

cyst
   aneurysmal bone c.
   bay c.
   branchial cleft c.
   buccal c.
   calcified radicular c.
   calcifying odontogenic c.
   central calcifying
      odontogenic c.
   cervical c.
   dental c.
   dental root c.
   dentigerous c.
   dentoalveolar c.
   dermoid c.
   developmental c's
   end root c.
   epidermoid c.
   eruption c.
   ganglion c.
   ghost cell odontogenic c.
   gingival c.
   gingival c. of the adult
   gingival c. of the newborn

cyst *(continued)*
    Gorlin c.
    hydatid c.
    implantation c.
    intraosseous calcifying
      odontogenic c.
    lateral periodontal c.
    lymphoepithelial c.
    maxillary c.
    median mandibular c.
    median palatal c.
    mucous duct c.
    nasoalveolar c.
    nasopalatine duct c.
    odontogenic c.
    oral heterotopic
      gastrointestinal c.
    orthokeratinized
      odontogenic c.
    paradental c.
    periapical c.

cyst *(continued)*
    periodontal c.
    primordial c.
    radicular c.
    residual c.
    residual periapical c.
    sialo-odontogenic c.
    synovial c.
    teratoid c.
    thyroglossal duct c.
    thyroglossal tract c.
    unicameral bone c.

cy·stat·in
    salivary c's

cys·tec·to·my

cy·to·meg·a·lo·vi·rus

Czer·mak
    C's line
    C's space

Dal·bo at·tach·ment

Dal·bo ex·tra·co·ro·nal at·tach·ment

Dal·bo ex·tra·co·ro·nal unit

Dal·bo stud at·tach·ment

Dal·bo stud unit

Dal·la Bo·na at·tach·ment

Dal·mane

Dal Pont
    Dal P. sagittal split
      osteotomy
    Obwegeser-D.P. sagittal
      split osteotomy

dam
    rubber d.

dam·age
    radiation d., soft tissue
    radiation d., teeth

Da·mas·cus disk

dam·mar

Dan·los
    Ehlers-D. syndrome

Dap·sone

Dar·by
    D.-Perry scaler

Da·rier
    D's disease

DAU
    Dental Auxiliary
      Utilization

Dau·ben·ton
    D's angle

Dau·trey
    D. operation

Da·vis
    D. crown
    D. root tip teaser

DCP
    dynamic compression plate

DDS
    Doctor of Dental Surgery

DDSc
    Doctor of Dental Science

Dean
    D. scissors

death
    pulp d.

de·band·ing

dé·bride·ment
    canal d.
    cavity d.
    chemical d.
    epithelial d.
    root canal d.

de·bris
    food d.

de·cay

de·cid·u·ous

de·con·ges·tant

dec·ta·flur

de·den·ti·tion

Dee-Eigh·teen gold al·loy

Dee·las·tic im·pres·sion ma·te·ri·al

Dee·one gold al·loy

Dee·pep-Hard gold al·loy

Dee·six gold al·loy

Dee·two gold al·loy

DEF
    decayed, extracted, filled
      (teeth)

de·fect
    dentoalveolar d.
    mandibular continuity d's
    marrow d.
    osteoporotic bone marrow
      d. of the mandible
    periodontal d.
    periodontal bony d.
    periodontal interradicular
      d.
    periodontal intrabony d.
    periodontal d. in marginal
      bone
    Stafne d.

De·fen·der pit and fis·sure
    seal·ant

de·fi·cien·cy
    condylar d.
    mandibular d.
    maxillary d.
    vertical d.
    vitamin d.

de·form·i·ty
    Andy Gump d.
    bird face d.
    craniofacial d's
    dentofacial d.
    facial d's
    Klippel-Feil d.

de·gas·sing

de·gen·er·a·tion
    atrophic pulp d.
    calcific pulp d.
    diffuse calcific pulp d.
    dystrophic pulp d.
    pulp d.

de·gen·er·a·tive

de·glov·ing

De·gu·fill H com·pos·ite

De·gu·fill M com·pos·ite

De·gu·flex im·pres·sion ma·te·
    ri·al

De·gu·flex Mono·phase poly·
    sil·ox·ane im·pres·sion
    ma·te·ri·al

de·his·cence
    alveolar d.
    root d.
    wound d.

Del·aire
    D. facemask

de Lange
    de L. syndrome

del·ta
    apical d.

Del·ta Den·tal Plan

Del·ton pit and fis·sure seal·
    ant

dem·e·clo·cy·cline

De·mer·ol

De·mer·ol HCl

De·nar ar·tic·u·la·tor

Den·holz
    D. appliance

dens *pl.* den·tes
    dentes acuti
    dentes decidui
    d. evaginatus
    dentes incisivi
    d. in dente
    d. invaginatus
    dentes molares
    dentes permanentes
    dentes premolares
    d. sapientiae
    d. serotinus

Den·sene 33 acryl·ic poly·mer

Dens·fil ob·tu·ra·tors

Dens·fil ther·mal en·do·don·
    tic ob·tu·ra·tors

den·si·ty
  bone d.

Den·stone den·tal stone

DENT
  Dental Exposure
    Normalization Technique

Den·ta·cam I in·tra·oral cam·era

Den·ta·cam II in·tra·oral cam·era

den·tag·ra

den·tal

Den·tal Aux·il·ia·ry Uti·li·za·tion (DAU)

Den·ta·leen

Den·tal Ex·po·sure Nor·mal·iza·tion Tech·nique (DENT)

Den·tal H top·i·cal flu·o·ride gel

Den·ta·lone

Den·tal Shade Com·par·a·tor

Dent·a·tus an·chor·age post

Dent·a·tus an·chor·age sys·tem

Dent·a·tus ar·tic·u·la·tor

den·tes

Dent Gold No. 1

Dent Gold No. 2

den·tia
  d. praecox
  d. tarda

den·ti·buc·cal

den·ti·cle
  adherent d.
  attached d.
  embedded d.
  false d.

den·ti·cle *(continued)*
  free d.
  interstitial d.
  true d.

den·ti·fi·ca·tion

den·ti·frice
  accepted d.
  fluoride d.
  monofluorophosphate d.
  provisionally accepted d.
  sodium fluoride d.
  stannous fluoride d.

den·tig·er·ous

den·ti·la·bi·al

den·ti·lin·gual

den·tim·e·ter

den·tin
  adventitious d.
  calcified d.
  circumpulpal d.
  d. cleaner
  coronal d.
  cover d.
  developmental d.
  functional d.
  hereditary opalescent d.
  interglobular d.
  intertubular d.
  irregular d.
  mantle d.
  opalescent d.
  peritubular d.
  primary d.
  radicular d.
  reparative d.
  residual carious d.
  sclerotic d.
  secondary d.
  secondary irregular d.
  secondary regular d.
  d. substitute
  tertiary d.
  transparent d.

Den·tin-Ac·ti·va·tor

den·ti·nal

den·tin·al·gia

den·tine

den·tin·i·fi·ca·tion

den·ti·no·blast

den·tino·clast

den·ti·no·gen·e·sis
    d. imperfecta

den·ti·no·gen·ic

den·ti·noid

den·ti·no·ma

Den·tin Pro·tec·tor

den·tist

den·tis·try
    ambulatory hospital d.
    ceramic d.
    community d.
    cosmetic d.
    dry field d.
    esthetic d.
    forensic d.
    four-handed d.
    geriatric d.
    group d.
    hospital d.
    industrial d.
    interceptive restorative d.
    legal d.
    operative d.
    outpatient hospital d.
    pediatric d.
    preventive d.
    primary care d.
    prophylactic d.
    prosthetic d.
    psychosomatic d.
    public health d.
    restorative d.
    seat-down d.
    solo d.
    stand-up d.
    team d.

den·tis·try *(continued)*
    TEAM d.
    washed field d.

den·ti·tion
    artificial d.
    deciduous d.
    delayed d.
    early mixed d.
    early permanent d.
    first d.
    mandibular d.
    maxillary d.
    mixed d.
    natural d.
    neonatal d.
    permanent d.
    precocious d.
    predeciduous d.
    premature d.
    primary d.
    retarded d.
    secondary d.
    temporary d.
    transitional d.

den·to·al·ve·o·lar

den·to·al·ve·o·li·tis

den·tode

den·to·fa·cial

den·to·form

den·tog·ra·phy

den·to·le·gal

Den·to·mat 3 Amal·ga·ma·tor

den·to·me·chan·i·cal

den·ton·o·my

den·to·sur·gi·cal

Den·tu-Creme

den·to·trop·ic

den·tu·lous

den·ture
    acrylic resin d.

den·ture *(continued)*
- d. adhesive
- articulated partial d.
- bar joint d.
- d. base
- base saddle d.
- broken-stress partial d.
- d. brush
- cantilever fixed partial d.
- clasp d.
- d. classification
- class I partial d.
- class II partial d.
- class III partial d.
- d. cleaner
- complete d.
- conditioning d.
- continuous gum d.
- d. curing
- distal extension d.
- distal extension partial d.
- duplicate d.
- d. edge
- esthetic d.
- d. esthetics
- extension partial d.
- fixed cantilever partial d.
- fixed partial d.
- d. flask
- full d.
- hinge d.
- immediate d.
- immediate-insertion d.
- implant d.
- interim d.
- Lee d.
- d. magnet
- metal base d.
- model wax d.
- mucosa-borne d.
- onlay d.
- overlay d.
- partial d.
- partial d., distal extension
- partial d., fixed
- partial d., removable
- partial d., unilateral
- periphery d.

den·ture *(continued)*
- polished surface d.
- precision d.
- precision retained d.
- d. prosthetics
- provisional d.
- removable d.
- removable partial d. (RPD)
- sectional partial d.
- d. sore mouth
- spoon d.
- d. stomatitis
- swing-lock d.
- telescopic d.
- temporary d.
- Ticonium hidden-lock d.
- tissue-borne d.
- tissue-borne partial d.
- tooth-borne d.
- tooth- and mucosa-borne d.
- transitional d.
- treatment d.
- trial d.
- unilateral partial d.

den·tur·ism

den·tur·ist

de·nu·da·tion
- interdental d.

Den·ver splint

de·pres·sion
- pterygoid d.
- tooth d.

de·pres·sor
- d. anguli oris
- d. labii inferioris

Derf
- D. needle holder

der·ma·to·fi·bro·ma

der·ma·to·fi·bro·sar·co·ma
- d. protuberans

der·moid

de·sen·si·tiz·er
  Zarosen d.

des·ig·na·tion
  Vita-Lumin shade d.

des·mo·don·ti·um

des·qua·ma·tive

de·torque

de·tor·sion

de·vel·op·ment
  dentofacial d.

de·vice
  acceptable d.
  Burnett ratchet d.
  central-bearing d.
  central-bearing tracing d.
  compression d.
  dynamic widening d's
  electronic root canal
    measuring d. (ERCM)
  Endoteck d.
  Joe Hall Morris external
    skeletal pin fixation d.
  provisionally acceptable d.
  Rota-dent plaque removal
    d.
  unacceptable d.

de·vi·tal·iza·tion
  pulp d.

de·vi·tal·ize

Dew·ey
  D. classification system

dex·a·meth·a·sone

Dex·on
  D. suture

di·a·be·tes

di·am·e·ter
  buccolingual d.
  labiolingual d. of crown
  labiolingual d. of crown at
    the cervix
  mesiodistal d. of crown

di·am·e·ter *(continued)*
  mesiodistal d. of crown at
    the cervix

dia·mond
  amalgam remover d.
  ball d.
  bulk reduction d.
  composite trimmer d.
  cone d.
  cone composite d.
  cone pointed d.
  cone round head d.
  contouring d.
  cylinder d.
  equilibrating d.
  flame d.
  flame composite d.
  flame finishing d.
  flame shape d.
  flat end cylinder d.
  flat end taper d.
  football d.
  gingival curettage d.
  gross reduction d.
  inverted cone d.
  multi-layered d.
  occlusal d.
  Omni operative d.
  operative d.
  Perio extra coarse d.
  pointed taper d.
  round d.
  round end taper d.
  silhouette d.
  straight cylinder flat end
  straight cylinder round
    end d.
  subgingival curettage d.
  superfine d.
  tapered cylinder–flat end
    d.
  tapered cylinder–round
    end d.
  wheel d.
  wheel round edge d.

di·a·phragm
  epithelial d.

di·a·stem

di·a·ste·ma *pl.* di·a·ste·ma·ta
 anterior d.

di·az·e·pam

di·a·zo·nal

di·a·zone

DIC
 disseminated intravascular
  coagulation

di·clo·fe·nac

di·clox·a·cil·lin

Di·cor MGC

DIC (dis·sem·i·nat·ed in·tra·
 vas·cu·lar co·ag·u·la·tion)
 syn·drome

die
 amalgam d.
 counter-d.
 electroformed d.
 electroplated d.
 plated d.
 d. stone
 waxing d.

Die Keen den·tal stone

Die·ker
 Miller-D. syndrome

Die Stone den·tal stone

di·eth·yl·di·thio·
 car·ba·mate

Di·George
 D. sequence

di·lac·er·a·tion

Di·lan·tin

di·men·sion
 contact vertical d.
 occlusal d.
 occlusal vertical d.
 postural vertical d.
 rest vertical d.

di·men·sion *(continued)*
 vertical d.
 vertical d., contact
 vertical d., postural
 vertical d., rest

diph·the·ria

di·phy·odont

DI-S
 simplified debris index

disc
 Sof-Lex contouring and
  polishing d's

dis·cec·to·my
 temporomandibular joint
  (TMJ) d.

dis·coid

dis·col·or·a·tion
 tooth d.

dis·co·plas·ty

dis·crep·an·cy
 arch length d.
 Bolton d.
 periodontal d.
 tooth size d.

dis·cus *pl.* dis·ci
 d. articularis articulationis
  mandibularis

dis·ease
 Addison's d.
 calcium pyrophosphate
  dihydrate crystal
  deposition d.
 cat-scratch d.
 CPPD crystal deposition d.
 Crohn's d.
 Cushing's d.
 Darier's d.
 Fauchard d.
 Gorham's d.
 graft-versus-host (GVH) d.
 hand-foot-and-mouth d.
 Hand-Schüller-Christian d.

dis·ease *(continued)*
  Heck's d.
  Hodgkin's d.
  idiopathic midline
    destructive d.
  Langerhans' cell d.
  Lyell's d.
  Mikulicz's d.
  Paget d.
  periodontal d.
  polycystic d.
  Riggs' d.
  von Willebrand's d.

dish
  dappen d.

dis·har·mo·ny
  occlusal d.

dis·junc·tion
  craniofacial d.

disk
  abrasive d.
  Burlew d.
  Carborundum d.
  cloth d.
  condylar d.
  cutting d.
  cuttlefish d.
  Damascus d.
  dental d.
  diamond d.
  emery d.
  Faskut abrasive d.
  finishing d.
  garnet d.
  Horico Diaflex diamond d.
  Jel-Thin 9 d.
  polishing d.
  safe-side d.
  sandpaper d.
  separating d.
  summa d.
  Super Snap buff d.
  Thin-Flex d.

dis·kec·to·my
  condylar d.

disk·ing

dis·ko·pexy
  condylar d.

dis·oc·clude

dis·or·der
  temporomandibular d.
    (TMD)

dis·pens·er
  mercury d.

Dis·per·sal·loy al·loy

dis·place·ment
  condylar d.

dis·tal

Dis·ta·lite com·pos·ite res·in

dis·tance
  cone d.
  cone-surface d.
  diaphragm-surface d.
  focal-film d.
  interarch d.
  interocclusal d.
  interridge d.
  long cone d.
  object-film d.
  short cone d.
  source-cone d.
  source-film d.
  source-surface d.
  target-film d.
  target-skin d.

dis·to·ax·io·gin·gi·val

dis·to·ax·io·in·ci·sal

dis·to·ax·io-oc·clu·sal

dis·to·buc·cal

dis·to·buc·co-oc·clu·sal

dis·to·buc·co·pul·pal

dis·to·cer·vi·cal

dis·to·cli·na·tion

dis·to·clu·sal

dis·to·clu·sion

dis·to·gin·gi·val

dis·to·la·bi·al

dis·to·la·bio·in·ci·sal

dis·to·lin·gual

dis·to·lin·guo·in·ci·sal

dis·to·lin·guo-oc·clu·sal

dis·to·lin·guo·pul·pal

dis·to·mo·lar

dis·to-oc·clu·sal

dis·to-oc·clu·sion

dis·to·place·ment

dis·to·pul·pal

dis·to·pul·po·la·bi·al

dis·to·pul·po·lin·gual

dis·to·ver·sion

dis·trac·tion

ditch·ing

di·ver·gence
    apical d.

di·vid·er
    stress d.

DLE
    discoid lupus
      erythematosus

DMB
    demineralized bone

DMB (demineralized bone)
    graft

DMF
    decayed, missing, filled
      (teeth)

DO
    disto-occlusal

DO (dis·to-oc·clu·sal) cav·i·ty

Doc·tor of Den·tal Sci·ence
    (DDSc)

Doc·tor of Den·tal Sur·gery
    (DDS)

Dr. Thomp·son's Col·or Trans·
    fer Ap·pli·ca·tors

Dol·der
    D. bar
    D. bar joint attachment
    D. bar unit
    D. bar unit attachment

dove·tail
    lingual d.
    occlusal d.

dow·el
    Thompson d.

Down
    D's analysis
    D. syndrome

down·frac·ture
    Le Fort I d.
    maxillary d.

down·graft
    chin d.
    maxillary d.

Downs
    D's Y axis

doxi·cy·cline

doxy·cy·cline

Doyle Air·way Splints

D-P Tra-Ten

drag

drain
    Penrose d.
    silicone d.

dress·ing
    absorbable collagen d.
    Alvogyl D.
    Barricaid VLC periodontal
      wound d.

dress·ing *(continued)*
    Chloro-Thymonol root
      canal d.
    Coe-Pak Automix
      periodontal d.
    CollaCote collagen wound
      d.
    CollaPlug collagen wound
      d.
    CollaTape collagen wound
      d.
    Colla-Tec absorbable
      collagen d.
    Cresanol root canal d.
    Getz Surgical D.
    M-C-P–root canal d.
    Periocare periodontal d.
    periodontal d.
    polyurethane d.
    pressure d.
    root canal d.
    semipermeable
      polyurethane d.

Dri-Aids

drift
    mesial d.
    physiologic d.

drift·ing
    tooth d.

drill
    bibeveled d.
    diamond d.
    double cutting d.
    Feldman d.
    Gates Glidden d.
    Micro-Vent double cutting
      d.
    Peeso d.
    Shannon d.
    spear-point d.
    twist d.

drill·ing

droop
    chin d.

drop
    Luride d's
    toothache d's

dro·per·i·dol

drop·let
    enamel d.

Drop·sin cal·ci·um hy·drox·ide

Drop·sin cal·ci·um hy·drox·ide
  base

drug
    nonsteroidal anti-
      inflammatory d.

Dry Guard Vi·ril·i·um Union
  Broach

D-type ream·er

Du·bo·witz
    D. syndrome

duct
    Bartholin's d.
    Blasius' d.
    parotid d.
    d's of Rivinus
    salivary d's
    Stensen's d.
    sublingual d's
    sublingual d., major
    sublingual d's, minor
    submandibular d.
    submaxillary d.
    Walther's d's
    Wharton's d.

Dum·bach Ti·ta·ni·um Mesh

Dum·bach ti·ta·ni·um plat·ing
  sys·tem

dum·my

Dun·lop
    Hirschfeld-D. file

Dunn
    Hart-D. attachment

Dun·ning
   D.-Leach index

Duo·mat 3 Amal·ga·ma·tor

Dura·fil re·stor·ative

Dura-Green den·tal stone

Du·ra·lay in·lay res·in

Du·ra Lin·er II

Du·ra·lon

Dur·al·loy al·loy

Dura-White den·tal stone

Du·re·lon car·box·yl·ate ce·ment

Du·re·lon ce·ment

Du·roc den·tal stone

Dutch gold

dwarf·ism
   pituitary d.

Dy·cal

Dy·cal ra·dio·paque cal·ci·um hy·drox·ide

dy·clo·nine

dye
   occlusal registration d.

dys·al·li·log·na·thia

dys·es·the·sia

dys·func·tion
   myofascial pain d.
   temporomandibular d.
   TMJ d.

dys·geu·sia

dys·ker·a·to·ma
   warty d.

dys·ker·a·to·sis
   d. congenita
   hereditary benign
      intraepithelial d.

dys·os·to·sis
   cleidocranial d.
   craniofacial d.

dys·pha·gia

dys·pla·sia
   anteroposterior facial d.
   camptomelic d.
   chondroectodermal d.
   cleidocranial d.
   condylar d.
   craniofacial fibrous d.
   dental d.
   dentin d., type I
   dentin d., type II
   dentoalveolar d.
   diastrophic d.
   ectodermal d's
   familial fibrous d.
   familial florid osseous d.
   familial osseous d.
   fibrous d.
   frontometaphyseal d.
   geleophysic d.
   hypohidrotic ectodermal d.
   Kniest d.
   Langer mesomelic d.
   maxillonasal d.
   monostotic fibrous d.
   osseous d.
   periapical cemental d.
   polyostotic fibrous d.
   Pyle metaphyseal d.
   spondyloepiphyseal d.
      congenita

dys·to·pia
   malar d.

Ea·gle
  E's syndrome
  E.-like syndrome

Eames
  E. technique

Ear·ly Pe·ri·od·ic Screen·ing Di·ag·no·sis Treat·ment (EPSDT)

EBA ce·ment

Eb·ner
  incremental line of E.
  line of E.

ebur
  e. dentis

Echi·no·coc·cus
  E. granulosus

Eclipse al·loy

ec·to·der·mal

ec·to·mes·en·chyme

EDA
  electronic dental
    anesthesia

ede·ma
  Berlin's e.

eden·tate

eden·tia

eden·tu·late

eden·tu·lous

edge
  beam e.
  bevel e.
  chamfer e.
  cutting e.
  denture e.
  incisal e.

edge-strength

edge·wise

Ed·lan
  E.-Mejchar procedure

EEC syn·drome

ef·fect
  bucket-handle e.
  chemotherapy e's
  fetal alcohol e's
  fetal aminopterin e's
  fetal hydantoin e's
  fetal rubella e's
  fetal trimethadione e's
  fetal valproate e's
  Karolyi e.
  maternal PKU fetal e's
  wedging e.

Ef·fer·dent

Eh·lers
  E.-Danlos syndrome

Ei·ken·el·la
  E. corrodens

ejec·tor
  apical fragment e.
  saliva e.

elas·tic
  class II e.
  class III e.
  interarch e.
  intermaxillary e.
  intramaxillary e.
  maxillomandibular e.
  rubber dam e.
  training e's
  vertical e.

Elas·ti·con

elas·to·mer

El·brecht
  E. splint

Elec·tra·loy

elec·trode
coagulating e.
fulgurating e.
gingival trough e.
incising e.
periodontia e.
tissue removal e.

elec·tro·form·er

elec·tro·mal·let
McShirley's e.

elec·tro·my·og·ra·phy

elec·tro·plat·ing

elec·tro·pol·ish·ing

elec·tro·ster·il·iza·tion
root canal e.

elec·tro·sur·gery

el·e·phan·ti·a·sis
e. gingivae

el·e·va·tor
Allen periosteal e.
angular e.
Apexo E.
apical e.
cross bar e.
Cryer e.
Cushing e.
dental e.
Goldman e.
Goldman-Fox periosteal e.
Henahan periosteal e.
Hu-Friedy E.
malar e.
Miller Apexo E.
Miller's e.
Molt e.
Molt periosteal e.
Ohl e.
periosteal e.
Potts' e.
Potts cross bar e.
Prichard periosteal e.
root e.

el·e·va·tor *(continued)*
root tip e.
Rowe zygomatic e.
screw e.
Seldin e.
Seldin periosteal e.
spear e.
straight e.
subperiosteal e.
T-bar e.
tooth e.
universal e.
wedge e.
West periosteal e.
Woodson e.

El·gi·loy

Elite ce·ment

elon·ga·tion
tooth e.

em·bra·sure
buccal e.
incisal e.
interdental e.
labial e.
lingual e.
occlusal e.

em·bry·op·a·thy
retinoic acid e.

em·ery

em·i·nec·to·my

em·i·nence
canine e.
e. of maxilla

em·i·nen·tia *pl.* em·i·nen·tiae
e. maxillae
e. symphysis

EMKA-Base glass ion·o·mer
ce·ment

EMKA-Fil glass ion·o·mer den·
tal re·stor·a·tive

EMKA glass ion·o·mer

EMKA re·stor·a·tive

EMKA-Sil·ver core ma·te·ri·al

EMKA-Sil·ver glass ion·o·mer
ce·ment

em·phy·se·ma
soft tissue e.

en·am·el
aprismatic e.
ceramic e.
e. cleaner
curled e.
dental e.
dwarfed e.
e. excrescence
e. fissure
gnarled e.
hereditary brown e.
hypoplastic e.
mottled e.
nanoid e.
opaque e.
e. spur
straight e.
white e.

Enam·el Etch·ant enam·el
prep

en·am·elo·blast

en·am·el·o·ma

enam·e·lo·plas·ty

end
distal e. of denture

end·ing
Ruffini's e's

En·do·ca·tor

en·do·don·tic

en·do·don·tics
pedodontic e.
surgical e.

en·do·don·tist

en·do·don·ti·um

en·do·don·tol·o·gist

en·do·don·tol·o·gy

en·do·don·to·ma

Endo-fill

en·do·gna·thi·on

En·do Ice re·frig·er·ant spray

En·do·me·ter

En·do·son·ic Dia·mond file

En·do·teck de·vice

En·do·teck spread·er

En·do·vage sy·ringe

en·flu·rane

en·gine
dental e.
high-speed e.
surgical e.
ultraspeed e.

En·hance fin·ish·ing and pol·
ish·ing sys·tem

en·large·ment
acute inflammatory
gingival e.
chronic inflammatory
gingival e.
combined gingival e.
diffuse gingival e.
discrete digingival e.
generalized gingival e.
gingival e.
inflammatory gingival e.
localized gingival e.
marginal gingival e.
papillary gingival e.
tumor-like gingival e.

epi·der·moid

epi·der·mol·y·sis
e. bullosa

epi·man·dib·u·lar

epi·neph·rine

ep·i·the·li·al

ep·i·the·li·um *pl.* ep·i·the·lia
  enamel e.
  gingival e.
  junctional e.
  sulcal e.
  sulcular e.

Epo·lene N-10 den·tal wax

Ep·oxy·lite 9070

Ep·oxy·lite 9075

EPSDT
  Early Periodic Screening
    Diagnosis Treatment

Ep·stein
  E's pearls

epu·lis *pl.* epu·li·des
  congenital e.
  e. fibromatosa
  e. fissurata
  giant cell e.
  e. gigantocellularis
  e. granulomatosa
  e. of newborn

ep·u·lo·fi·bro·ma

ep·u·loid

equal·iz·er
  Ballard stress e.
  stress e.

equa·tion
  Bancroft e.

equi·li·bra·tion
  mandibular e.
  occlusal e.

ERCM
  electronic root canal
    measuring device

Erich
  E. arch bar

ero·sion
  dental e.

ero·sion *(continued)*
  dish-shaped e.
  notch-shaped e.
  saucer-shaped e.
  V-shaped e.
  wedge-shaped e.

ero·sive

erup·tion
  active e.
  altered passive e.
  continuous e.
  delayed e.
  delayed passive e.
  ectopic e.
  forced e.
  passive e.
  premature e.
  surgical e.
  tooth e.

erup·tive

er·y·the·ma
  e. migrans
  e. multiforme

er·y·them·a·to·sus

eryth·ro·blas·to·sis
  e. fetalis, e.

Eryth·ro·cin

eryth·ro·my·cin
  e. acistrate

eryth·ro·pla·kia

Es·co·bar
  E. syndrome

Es·pe Ro·ca·tec-Sys·tem

Es·sig
  E.-type splint
  E.-type splinting

Es·the·lite

es·thet·ic

Es·the·ti·Cone

es·the·tics
 automated e.
 denture e.
 natural e.

Es·ti·lux Pos·te·ri·or com·pos·
 ite res·in

Est·lan·der
 Abbe-E. flap

etch
 Onyx L/G Black E.

etch·ant
 Herculite XR gel e.

etch·ing
 acid e.

Etch N' Seal

Etch Pro·tect

Eth·i·con su·tures

Eu·bac·te·ri·um

eu·ca·lyp·tol

eu·ca·per·cha

eu·gen·ic acid

eu·gen·ol

eu·gna·thia

eu·gnath·ic

eu·ryg·nath·ic

eu·ryg·na·thism

eva·gi·na·tus

Ev·ans
 E. articulator

Ev·er·best Pro·son·ic den·ture
 cleans·er

EVRO
 extraoral vertical ramus
 osteotomy

Ew·ing
 E's sarcoma

Exac·ta-Film ar·tic·u·lat·ing
 film

Ex·a·flex im·pres·sion ma·te·
 ri·al

Ex·a·mix im·pres·sion ma·te·
 ri·al

ex·ca·va·tion
 dental e.

ex·ca·va·tor
 dental e.
 hatchet e.
 spoon e.

ex·ce·men·to·sis

ex·cess
 mandibular e.
 maxillary e.
 vertical e.

ex·cur·sion
 lateral e.
 left lateral e.
 protrusive e.
 retrusive e.
 right lateral e.

ex·cur·sive

ex·er·cis·er
 jaw e's
 Therabite personal e.

ex·fo·li·a·tive

ex·odon·tia

ex·odon·tics

ex·odon·tist

ex·og·e·nous

ex·og·na·thia

ex·og·na·thi·on

ex·os·to·sis
 osteocartilaginous
 exostoses

ex·pan·der
 graft e.

ex·pan·der *(continued)*
    rapid intraoperative tissue
      e. (RITE)
    subperiosteal tissue e.
      (STE)
    tissue e.

ex·pan·sion
    e. of the arch
    cubical e.
    delayed e.
    effective setting e.
    hygroscopic e.
    hygroscopic setting e.
    maxillary e.
    mercuroscopic e.
    normal setting e.
    palatal e.
    rapid maxillary e. (RME)
    rapid palatal e. (RPE)
    secondary e.
    setting e.
    slow maxillary e.
    thermal e.
    transverse e.
    wax e.

ex·plor·er
    cowhorn e.
    dental e.
    double end e.
    Expros e./probe
    Glick e.
    "pig tail" e.
    root canal e.
    single end e.

ex·po·sure
    keratopathy e.

Ex·press bite reg·is·tra·tion
    ma·te·ri·al

Ex·press im·pres·sion ma·te·
    ri·al

Ex·pros ex·plor·er/probe

ex·ten·sion
    groove e.
    e. for prevention
    ridge e.

ex·ter·nal

ex·tir·pa·tion
    dental pulp e.

ex·tra·buc·cal

ex·tra·cap·su·lar

ex·tract

ex·trac·tion
    elevator e.
    flap e.
    forceps e.
    painless e.
    rubber band e.
    progressive e.
    selected e.
    serial e.
    tooth e.

ex·trac·tor

ex·tra·den·tal

ex·tra·oral

ex·tra·ver·sion

ex·tro·ver·sion

ex·trude

Ex·trude Ex·tra im·pres·sion
    ma·te·ri·al

Ex·trude im·pres·sion ma·te·
    ri·al

ex·tru·sion
    vertical e.

ex·u·vi·a·tion

eye·let

E-Z Flap

Fa·bry
    F's syndrome

face
    dolichocephalic f.

face-bow
    adjustable axis f.-b.
    arbitrary f.-b.
    Hanau f.-b.
    kinematic f.-b.
    preformed f.-b.
    f.-b. record

face·mask
    Delaire f.

face·om·e·ter

fac·er
    root f.

fac·et
    occlusal f.

fa·cial

fa·ci·es *pl.* fa·ci·es
    adenoid f.
    f. anterior dentium
        premolarium et molarium
    f. articularis fossae
        mandibularis
    balloon f.
    f. buccalis dentis
    f. labialis dentis
    f. lateralis dentium
        incisivorum et caninorum
    f. masticatoria dentis
    f. medialis dentium
        incisivorum et caninorum
    f. posterior dentium
        premolarium et molarium

fac·ing
    interchangeable f.
    Steele's f.

fa·cio·ste·no·sis

fac·tor
    bone f.

fas·cia *pl.* fas·ciae
    f. parotideomasseterica
    f. temporalis

fas·ci·cle

Fas·kut abra·sive disk

Fas·tray

fa·tigue
    material f.

fat pad
    buccal f.p.

Fau·chard
    F. disease

FDI
    Fédération Dentaire
    Internationale

Fé·dé·ra·tion Den·taire In·ter·
na·tio·nale (FDI)

Feil
    Klippel-F. deformity
    Klippel-F. sequence

Feld·man
    F. bur
    F. drill

feld·spar
    calcium f.
    potassium f.
    soda f.
    sodium f.

fen·es·tra·tion
    alveolar plate f.
    apical f.

fen·ta·nyl

fen·ta·nyl cit·rate

Fer·gus·son
    F's incision

Fer·gus·son *(continued)*
    Weber-F. incision
    F's operation

Fer·mit com·pos·ite res·in

Fer·rein
    F's ligament

Fer·ri·er
    F. 212 gingival clamp
    F's separator

fes·toon
    gingival f.
    McCall's f.

fes·toon·ing

fe·tal·is

fe·tor
    f. ex ore
    f. oris

fi·ber
    alveolar f's
    alveolar crest f's
    apical f's
    argyrophilic f's
    C f's
    cemental f's
    cementoalveolar f's
    circular f's
    circular gingival f's
    collagen f's
    definite f's
    dentinal f.
    dentinogenic f's
    depressor f's
    elastic f's
    gingival f's
    gingival f's, transseptal
    gingivodental f's
    horizontal f's
    intergingival f's
    intermediate f's
    interradicular f's
    Korff f's
    oblique f's
    odontogenic f's
    perforating f's

fi·ber *(continued)*
    principal f's
    semicircular f's
    Sharpey's f's
    supracrestal f.
    Tomes f.
    tooth attachment f's
    transseptal f's

Fi·ber-Pink Acryl·ic Res·in

Fi·ber-Pink Tri·ad Res·in

fi·bril
    anchoring f.
    dentinal f's
    Tomes f.

fi·bril·lo·blast

fi·bro·chon·dro·gen·e·sis

fi·bro·epi·the·li·al

fi·bro·ma
    ameloblastic f.
    cemento-ossifying f.
    central odontogenic f.
    central ossifying f.
    desmoplastic f.
    giant cell f.
    granular cell ameloblastic
        f.
    granular cell odontogenic f.
    juvenile ossifying f.
    odontogenic f.
    ossifying f.
    ossifying f., peripheral
    peripheral odontogenic f.
    peripheral ossifying f.

fi·bro·ma·to·sis
    aggressive f.
    f. gingivae
    gingival f.
    idiopathic gingival f.

fi·bro·myo·sar·co·ma
    f. of the nerve

fi·bro·myx·o·ma
    odontogenic f.

fi·bro·nec·tin

fi·bro-odon·to·ma
    ameloblastic f.

fi·bro-os·te·o·ma
    central f.

fi·bro·sar·co·ma
    ameloblastic f.
    neurogenic f.
    odontogenic f.
    well-differentiated f.

fi·bro·sis
    intra-articular f.
    oral submucous f.
    pulp f.
    subepidermal nodular f.
    submucous f.

fi·bro·to·my
    circumferential
        supracrestal f.

fi·brous

field
    dry f.

file
    bone f.
    endodontic f.
    Endosonic Diamond f.
    engine f.
    finishing f.
    Flex-R f.
    Giro f.
    gold f.
    Hedström f.
    Hirschfeld f.
    Hirschfeld-Dunlop f.
    Howard f.
    H-type f.
    H-type root canal f.
    Kerr f.
    K-Flex f.
    K-type root canal f.
    Miller-Colburn f.
    Orban f.
    periodontal f.
    rat-tail f.

file *(continued)*
    root canal f.
    rubber f.
    S f.
    scaler f.
    Schluger f.
    Star root canal f.
    Sugarman f.
    vulcanite f.

fil·ing

fill·er
    Giro spiral f's
    Lentulo spiral paste f's
    paste f's
    resin f.

fill·ing
    bead technique f.
    brush technique f.
    complex f.
    composite f.
    compound f.
    direct f.
    direct resin f.
    ditched f.
    flow technique f.
    indirect f.
    f. material
    Mosetig-Moorhof f.
    permanent f.
    postresection f.
    pressure technique f.
    retrograde f.
    reverse f.
    root canal f.
    root-end f.
    temporary f.
    treatment f.

Fil·Lock ream·er

film
    Accu Film articulating f.
    Articu-Film articulating f.
    bite-wing f.
    dental f's
    Exacta-Film articulating f.
    extraoral f.

film *(continued)*
    intraoral f.
    laminagraphic f.
    occlusal f.
    periapical f.
    ultraspeed radiographic f.

Fil·pin sys·tem

Fil·post

Fi·nesse re·stor·a·tive

fin·ish·ing
    interdental f.

fir·ing
    air f.
    diffusible gas f.
    high biscuit f.
    high bisque f.
    low biscuit f.
    medium biscuit f.
    medium bisque f.
    pressure f.
    vacuum f.

Fir·mi·lay al·loy

Fisch·er
    F. pliers

fis·su·ra·tum

fis·sure
    maxillary f.
    oral f.
    retrocuticular f.
    f. sealant

fis·tu·la *pl.* fis·tu·lae, fis·tu·las
    alveolar f.
    lateral palatal f's
    nasolabial f.
    oroantral f.
    oronasal f.
    salivary f.

fit
    marginal f.
    passive f.

FITC
    fluorescein isothiocyanate

Fit Check·er

F.I.T.T. func·tion·al im·pres·sion tis·sue ton·er

fix·a·tion
    biphasic pan f.
    circumalveolar f.
    circumpalatal f.
    craniomaxillary f.
    elastic band f.
    external pin f.
    intermaxillary f.
    internal f.
    jaw f.
    mandibulomaxillary f.
    maxillomandibular f.
    microplate f.
    miniplate f.
    monocortical plate f.
    nasomandibular f.
    palatal screw f.
    rigid internal f. (RIF)
    screw f.
    semirigid f.
    titanium mesh f.

Flag·yl

flange
    buccal f.
    denture f.
    labial f.
    lingual f.
    mandibular lingual f.

flap
    Abbe-Estlander f.
    Bakamijam f.
    bicoronal f.
    bipedicled f.
    cervical f.
    deltopectoral f.
    envelope f.
    E-Z F.
    full thickness periodontal f.
    intrasulcular f.

flap *(continued)*
    Langenbeck's pedicle
      mucoperiosteal f.
    lingual tongue f.
    L-shaped septal
      chondromucosal f's
    Luebke-Ochsenbein f.
    microvascular free f.
    modified Widman f.
    mucoperiosteal f.
    mucoperiosteal periodontal
      f.
    mucosal periodontal f.
    myocutaneous f.
    myocutaneous pedicled f.
    osteomyocutaneous f.
    partial thickness
      periodontal f.
    pedicled
      osteomyocutaneous f.
    periodontal f.
    pharyngeal f's
    simple periodontal f.
    skin f's
    sternocleidomastoid f.
    von Langenbeck's bipedicle
      mucoperiosteal f.
    Widman f.
    Widman f., modified

flare
    alar f.

flash

flask
    casting f.
    crown f.
    denture f.
    injection f.
    molding f.
    refractory f.

flask·ing

Flecks ce·ment

Fleisch·mann
    F's bursa
    F's follicle

Flex·acryl re·base acryl·ic

Flex·i·con im·pres·sion ma·
    te·ri·al

Flexi-Flow com·pos·ite ce·
    ment

Flexi-Post over·den·ture

Flexi-Post ream·er

Flex·o·files

Flex·o·wax C

Flex-R file

FLH
    follicular lymphoid
      hyperplasia

floss
    dental f.

floss·ing

flour
    f. of pumice

flow

Flow·er
    F's index

Flow-Temp ce·ment

flu·co·na·zole

flu·id
    dentinal f.

flu·o·res·cein iso·thio·cy·a·
    nate (FITC)

flu·o·ride
    stannous f.

Flu·o·ri·dent li·quid

Flu·o·ro·Core Build-up Sys·
    tem

Flu·o·ro·Core core ma·te·ri·al

Flu·or-O-Kote top·i·cal flu·o·
    ride gel

Flu·o·ro·shield pit and fis·sure
    seal·ant

Flu·o·ro·shield pit and fis·sure
    seal·ant

flu·o·ro·sis
    dental f.
    endemic f., chronic

Flu·o·ro-Thin ce·ment

5-flu·o·ro·ura·cil

flu·phen·a·zine

flur·az·e·pam

flur·bip·ro·fen

flux
    casting f.
    ceramic f.
    neutral f.
    oxidizing f.
    reducing f.
    soldering f.

FMA trans·la·tor

foil
    f. assistant
    f. carrier
    cohesive gold f.
    f. condenser
    corrugated gold f.
    gold f.
    gold f., cohesive
    gold f. condensation
    f. holder
    invisible f.
    laminated gold f.
    mat f.
    noncohesive gold f.
    f. passer
    f. pellet
    platinized f.
    platinum f.
    f. plugger
    f. rope
    semicohesive gold f.
    tin f.
    tin f. substitute

fold
    mucobuccal f.
    mucolabial f.
    mucosobuccal f.

fold *(continued)*
    palatine f's
    transverse palatine f's

fol·li·cle
    dental f.
    Fleischmann's f.
    tooth f.

Fones
    F. method of toothbrushing

fo·ra·men *pl.* fo·ra·mi·na
    accessory f.
    dental foramina
    lateral f.
    maxillary f., anterior
    maxillary f., internal
    maxillary f., posterior
    pulpal f.
    f. radicis dentis
    root f.

Forbes
    F. disease

force
    anchorage f.
    bite f.
    biting f.
    chewing f.
    compressive f.
    condensing f.
    constant f.
    denture-dislodging f.
    denture-retaining f.
    differential f.
    differential orthodontic f.
    extraoral f.
    masticatory f.
    maximal biting f.
    occlusal f.
    optimum orthodontic f.
    orthodontic f.
    reciprocal f.
    tooth-moving f.

for·ceps
    Adson f.
    Adson-Brown f.
    alligator f.

for·ceps *(continued)*
 Allis tissue f.
 Allison f.
 apical fragment f.
 articulating paper f.
 Asch f.
 bayonet f.
 Brewer's f.
 bulldog f.
 bullet f.
 chalazion f.
 clamp f.
 clip f.
 corn suture f.
 cow horn f.
 Cryer f.
 dental f.
 dressing f.
 extracting f.
 fixation f.
 horn beak f.
 Hu-Friedy f.
 Ivory f.
 Ivory rubber dam clamp f.
 Kazanjian f.
 L f.
 Laborde's f.
 Liston's f.
 lock f.
 Löwenberg's f.
 MaGill f.
 mandibular f.
 mandibular anterior teeth
  f.
 mandibular molar f.
 mandibular posterior f.
 mandibular third molar f.
 maxillary bicuspid f.
 maxillary incisor f.
 maxillary molar f.
 maxillary premolar f.
 f. MD3
 f. MD4
 f. Mead 3
 f. Mead 4
 microsurgical f.
 mosquito f.
 Nevius f.

for·ceps *(continued)*
 f. No. 16
 f. No. 18
 f. No. 24
 f. No. 88
 f. No. 99-A
 f. No. 99-C
 f. No. 103
 f. No. 150
 f. No. 151
 f. No. 222
 f. No. 286
 f. No. 287
 pedo f.
 point f.
 R f.
 rongeur f.
 Rowe maxillary
  disimpaction f.
 rubber dam f.
 rubber dam clamp f.
 Semken-Taylor f.
 silver point f's
 splinter f.
 splitting f.
 Stieglitz fragment and root
  f.
 suture f.
 tenaculum f.
 Tessier f.
 thumb f.
 tissue f.
 tongue f.
 torsion f.
 universal f.
 universal cow horn f.
 University of Washington
  rubber dam clamp f.
 Walsham f.

For·dyce
 F's granules

fo·ren·sic

form
 anatomic f.
 arch f.
 Brader arch f.

form *(continued)*
  occlusal f.
  Osteo-Loc plate f.
  Osteo-Loc root f.
  outline f.
  resistance f.
  retention f.
  spherical f. of occlusion
  strip-off crown f's
  tooth f.
  uniform report f.

for·ma·tion
  buttressing bone f.
  pseudodisk f.

For·ma·tray

For·ma·tron IV Dig·i·tal apex lo·ca·tor

form·er
  angle f.
  crucible f.
  glass f.
  sprue f.

for·mo·cre·sol

for·mu·la *pl.* for·mu·lae, for·mu·las
  Black's f. (for identifying handcutting instruments)
  dental f.
  four-number f.

For·ti·cast al·loy

fos·sa *pl.* fos·sae
  digastric f.
  glenoid f.
  incisive f. of maxilla
  maxillary f.
  f. musculi biventeris
  mylohyoid f. of mandible
  myrtiform f.
  f. praenasalis
  prenasal f.
  pterygoid f. of inferior maxillary bone
  sublingual f.
  submandibular f.

fos·sa *(continued)*
  submaxillary f.

Fos·sa-Em·i·nence pros·the·sis

foun·da·tion
  ADA Health F.
  denture f.

fo·vea *pl.* fo·veae
  f. of condyloid process
  digastric f.

Fox
  F. scissors
  F.-Williams probe
  Goldman-F. curet
  Goldman-F. knife
  Goldman-F. nipper
  Goldman-F. periosteal elevator
  Goldman-F. probe
  Goldman-F. scaler
  Goldman-F. scissors
  Goldman-F. spear knife

frac·ture
  avulsive f.
  condylar f.
  craniofacial f's
  crown f.
  Guérin's f.
  horizontal maxillary f.
  Jefferson f.
  Le Fort's f.
  mandibular f.
  midface f's
  odontoid f.
  orbital blowout f.
  pyramidal f. (of maxilla)
  ramus f's
  teardrop f.
  tetrapod f's
  transverse facial f.
  transverse maxillary f.
  tripod f.

frac·ture-dis·lo·ca·tion
  mandibular f.-d.

frag·ment
    condylar f.

frame
    halo head f.
    head f.
    Nygaard-Otsby f.
    occluding f.
    Otsby f.
    peripheral subperiosteal f.
    radiolucent f.
    ramus f.
    rubber dam f.
    superstructure f.
    Wizard f.
    Young f.

frame·work
    implant f.

Frän·kel
    F. appliance

Frank·fort Hor·i·zon·tal

Frank·fort Hor·i·zon·tal line

Frank·fort Hor·i·zon·tal plane

Frank·fort–man·dib·u·lar
    plane an·gle

Fra·ser
    F. syndrome

Fra·zier
    F. aspirator

Free·man
    F.-Sheldon syndrome

French chalk

French spring eye nee·dle

fre·nec·to·my
    flap f.

fre·not·o·my
    lingual f.

fren·u·lum pl. fren·u·la
    f. of inferior lip
    f. linguae
    f. of superior lip

fren·u·lum (continued)
    f. of tongue

fre·num pl. fre·na
    buccal f.
    labial f.
    f. labiorum
    lingual f.
    f. of tongue

Frey
    F's syndrome

Fried·man
    F. splint
    mini-F. rongeur

frit

frit·ting

fruc·to·fu·ra·nose

fruc·tose-6-phos·phate

Fu·ji Cap II re·stor·ative

Fu·ji Lin·ing glass ion·o·mer
    ce·ment

Fu·ji Lin·ing LC ce·ment

Fu·ji I lut·ing ce·ment

Fu·ji II glass ion·o·mer re·stor
    ·ative

Fu·ji II LC glass ion·o·mer re·
    stor·ative

Fu·ji II re·stor·ative

Fu·ji·rock den·tal stone

Ful-Fil com·pos·ite res·in

Ful-Fil re·stor·a·tive

fu·ma·rate
    ferrous f.

fun·goides

fur·ca pl. fur·cae

fur·cal

fur·ca·tion

fur·ca·tion·plas·ty

Fur·low
    F. double Z-plas·ty

fur·nace
    inlay f.

fu·ro·se·mide

Fu·sion
    centric f.
    latent heat of f.

Fu·sion *(continued)*
    tandem f.
    tooth f.

Fu·so·bac·te·ri·um
    F. nucleatum

fu·so·bac·te·ri·um *pl.* fu·so·
    bac·te·ria

fu·so·spi·ril·lo·sis

Fy·nal ce·ment

Gaer·ny
G. bar

gag
Molt mouth g.
g. reflex

ga·lac·to·py·ra·nose

gan·gli·on *pl.*gan·glia, gan·gli·
ons
gasserian g.
semilunar g.

gan·o·blast

gap
interocclusal g.

Gard·ner
G's syndrome

gar·net

Gar·ré
G's osteomyelitis

Gates
Gow-G. mandibular block

Gates Glid·den bur

Gates Glid·den drill

gauge
Boley g.
BW g.
depth g.
Johnichi torque g.
modified Boley g. (MBG)
Starret wire g.
test file g.
undercut g.

gauze
iodoform g.

gear
cervical g.
head g.

gel
acidulated phosphate
fluoride (APF) g.
aluminum hydroxide g.
benzocaine g.
Coe Hydrophilic G.
Etch g.
Gel-Tin fluoride g.
Kerr topical Flura-G.
Nupro APF g.
Nupro fluoride g.
PerioSELECT fluoride g.
Peroxyl g.
phosphoric acid g.
Scotchbond etching g.
60 Second Taste Fluoride
G.
sodium fluoride and
orthophosphoric acid g.
SofScale calculus scaling g.
Spring White 10 whitening
g.
Stan-Gard fluoride g.
Thixo-Gel fluoride g.
Topex 00:60 fluoride g.
Topicale anesthetic g.
Triad g.

Gel-Etch

Gel·film

Gel-Tain·er

Gel-Tin flu·o·ride gel

gem·i·na·tion

gen·er·a·tor
x-ray g.

ge·nio·plas·ty
advancement g.

ge·ni·ot·o·my
high sliding horizontal g.

gen·ta·mi·cin
g. sulfate

Ger·ber
G. space maintainer

ger·i·at·rics
dental g.

geri·odon·tics

geri·odon·tist

Ge·ri·stone Com·pos·ite

Ge·ri·store ad·he·sive res·in

germ
dental g.
enamel g.
tooth g.

ger·odon·tia

ger·odon·tic

ger·odon·tics

ger·odon·tist

ger·odon·tol·o·gy

Getz den·tin con·di·tion·er

Getz Sur·gi·cal Dress·ing

GI
gingival index

Gied·i·on
Langer-G. syndrome
Schinzel-G. syndrome

gi·gan·tism

Gil·lies
G. method
G. operation

Gil·mer
G's splint
G. wiring

Gil·son
G. fixable-removable bar

Gin·gi·caine

Gin·gi·pak re·trac·tion cord

gin·gi·va *pl.* gin·gi·vae
alveolar g.

gin·gi·va *(continued)*
areolar g.
attached g.
buccal g.
cemental g.
free g.
interdental g.
interproximal g.
labial g.
lingual g.
marginal g.
papillary g.
septal g.
unattached g.

gin·gi·val

gin·gi·val·gia

gin·gi·val·ly

gin·gi·vec·to·my

gin·gi·vi·tis
acute necrotizing
ulcerative g. (ANUG)
acute ulcerative g.
acute ulceromembranous
g.
atrophic senile g.
catarrhal g.
cotton-roll g.
desquamative g.
Dilantin g.
eruptive g.
fusospirochetal g.
g. gravidarum
hemorrhagic g.
herpetic g.
hormonal g.
hyperplastic g.
marginal g.
marginal g., generalized
marginal g., simple
g. marginalis suppurativa
necrotizing ulcerative g.
papillary g.
phagedenic g.
plasma cell g.
pregnancy g.

gin·gi·vi·tis *(continued)*
    streptococcal g.
    suppurative g.
    tuberculous g.
    Vincent's g.

gin·gi·vo·buc·co·ax·i·al

gin·gi·vo·la·bi·al

gin·gi·vo·lin·guo·ax·i·al

gin·gi·vo·peri·odon·ti·tis
    necrotizing ulcerative g.

gin·gi·vo·plas·ty

gin·gi·vo·sis

gin·gi·vo·sto·ma·ti·tis
    herpetic g.

Gi·rard
    Carroll-G. screw

Gi·ro en·gine ream·ers

Gi·ro Files

Gi·ro·mat·ic hand·piece

Gi·ro spi·ral fill·ers

gla·bel·la

gland
    admaxillary g.
    buccal g's
    cheek g's
    genal g's
    gingival g's
    glossopalatine g's
    labial g's of mouth
    malar g's
    mandibular g.
    g's of mouth
    parotid g.
    parotid g., accessory
    Rivinus g.
    salivary g's
    salivary g., external
    salivary g., internal
    salivary g's, major
    salivary g's, minor
    sublingual g.

gland *(continued)*
    submandibular g.
    submaxillary g.
    Suzanne's g.

glan·du·la *pl.* glan·du·lae
    g. incisiva
    glandulae oris
    g. parotidea
    g. parotidea accessoria
    g. submandibularis

glan·du·lar·is

Glas·Ion·o·mer ce·ment

glass
    g. former
    g. ionomer cement
    leaded g.
    Pyrex g.
    g. transition temperature
    Vycor G.

Glas·stone den·tal stone

glaze
    high g.
    low g.
    medium g.

Glick
    G. explorer

Glick·man
    G. probe
    G. scissors

glide
    mandibular g.
    occlusal g.

gli·o·ma
    malignant peripheral g.

glo·bo·don·tia

glos·sec·to·my

glos·si·tis
    median rhomboid g.

glos·so·dyn·ia

glos·so·pha·ryn·ge·al

glos·so·plas·ty

glos·sor·rha·phy

glos·so·ster·e·sis

glos·sot·o·my
    midline sagittal g.

Glos·sy pol·ish·ing paste

glu·cose
    g. 1-phosphate
    g. 6-phosphate

glue
    dermal g.

Glu·ma bond·ing sys·tem

Glu·ma 3-Step bond·ing sys·tem

glyc·er·in
    anhydrous g.

glyc·er·ol

glyc·er·yl
    g. tristearate

gly·co·ca·lyx

gly·cos·ami·no·gly·can

GMS
    Gomoramine methenamine
        silver (stains)

GMT
    gingival margin trimmer

gnatho·dy·nam·ics

gnatho·dy·na·mom·e·ter
    bimeter g.

gnath·og·ra·phy

gnatho·log·ic

gnath·ol·o·gy

gnatho·plas·ty

gnatho·stat·ics

Goe·the
    suture of G.

gold
    Aderer No. 3 Bridge G.
    Aleco g. alloy
    Aleco No. 4 g. alloy
    Aleco No. 5 g. alloy
    Aleco No. 9 g. alloy
    g. alloy
    g. amalgam
    American G. "B" Bridge
    American G. "C" Partial
        Extra Hard
    American G. "M-H" inlay
    American G. "M" inlay
        medium
    American G. "T" Bridge
        Hard
    annealed g.
    Bridge III-C g. alloy
    Bridge Partial IV-D g.
        alloy
    g. bromide
    24 carat g.
    cohesive g.
    cohesive g. foil
    colloidal g.
    g.-copper system
    Crown Hylastic g. alloy
    Crown Knapp No. 3 g.
        alloy
    Crown No. 1 g. alloy
    Crown No. 3 g. alloy
    Crown Supreme g. alloy
    Crown TT g. alloy
    Dee-Eighteen g. alloy
    Deeone g. alloy
    Deepep-Hard g. alloy
    Deesix g. alloy
    Deetwo g. alloy
    dental g.
    Dent G. No. 1
    Dent G. No. 2
    direct g.
    direct filling g.
        condensation
    Dutch g.
    electrolytic g.
    encapsulated powdered g.
    1000 fine g.

gold *(continued)*
  g. foil
  g. foil condensation
  Goldent powdered g.
  g. inlay
  Jelenko No. 7 g. alloy
  g. knife
  mat g.
  MF-Y g.
  Mowrey 120 g. alloy
  Mowrey No. 8 g. alloy
  Mowrey S-1 g. alloy
  Mowrey S-3 g. alloy
  noncohesive g.
  noncohesive g. foil
  Nürnberg g.
  g. plating
  platinized g.
  g. plugger
  powdered g.
  pure g.
  radioactive g.
  g. sodium thiomalate
  g. sodium thiosulfate
  g. solder
  sponge g.
  Sterngold 1 g. alloy
  Sterngold 2 g. alloy
  Sterngold 3 g. alloy
  Sterngold 5 g. alloy
  Sterngold B g. alloy
  Sterngold S g. alloy
  Sterngold Supercast g.
    alloy
  g. thioglucose
  white g.
  yellow g.

Gol·den·har
  G. hemifacial microsomia

Gol·dent pow·dered gold

Gold·ies car·bide burs

Gold·link Opa·quer

Gold·man
  G. elevator
  G.-Fox curet

Gold·man *(continued)*
  G.-Fox knife
  G.-Fox nipper
  G.-Fox periosteal elevator
  G.-Fox probe
  G.-Fox scaler
  G.-Fox scissors
  G.-Fox spear knife

Gold·smith
  G. I inlay

Goltz
  G. syndrome

Go·mor·amine meth·en·amine
  sil·ver stains

gon·or·rhea

Goode
  Younger-G. curet
  Younger-G. scaler

Gor·don
  G. pliers

Gore-Tex aug·men·ta·tion ma·
  te·ri·al

Gore-Tex re·gen·er·a·tive ma·
  te·ri·al

Gor·ham
  G's disease

Gor·lin
  G. cyst
  G. syndrome

Gos·lee
  G. tooth

Goth·ic arch trac·ing

Gow
  G.-Gates mandibular block

Gra·cey
  G. curet

graft
  AAA (autolyzed antigen-
    extracted allogeneic) g.
  allogeneic g.

graft *(continued)*
    autogenous g.
    bone g's
    cancellous bone g's
    composite g's
    condylar g.
    cortical bone g's
    corticocancellous bone g's
    costochondral g's
    costochondral onlay g's
    crib g.
    demineralized bone g.
    dermal g.
    double papilla pedicle g.
    endochondral bone g.
    free gingival g.
    full thickness mucosal g.
    full thickness periodontal
      g.
    gingival g.
    iliac g.
    interpositional bone g's
    intramembranous bone g's
    labiobuccal g's
    L-shaped iliac crest bone g.
    mucoperiosteal periodontal
      g.
    mucosal g.
    mucosal periodontal g.
    onlay g.
    palatal g's
    papillary pedicle g.
    partial thickness
      periodontal g.
    particulate bone g.
    pedicle g.
    periosteal g.
    resorbable bone g.
    rib g.
    skin g.
    split thickness g.
    split thickness periodontal
      g.

Grang·er
    G. articulator

gran·ule
    Fordyce's g's

gran·ule *(continued)*
    keratohyaline g's

gran·u·lo·ma *pl.* gran·u·lo·
  mas, gran·u·lo·ma·ta
    apical g.
    central giant cell g.
    dental g.
    eosinophilic g.
    eosinophilic g. of mandible
    g. gangrenescens
    giant cell g's
    malignant g.
    midline lethal g.
    periapical g.
    peripheral giant cell g's
    pyogenic g.
    radicular g.
    traumatic g.

gran·u·lo·ma·to·sa

gran·u·lo·ma·to·sis
    Wegener's g.

grasp
    modified pen g.
    palm and thumb g.
    pen g.

gra·vis

Greene
    G.-Vermillion index

Green·ie den·tal stone

Gregg
    G. filling instrument

Grey Com·pound

Grif·fin
    G. appliance

grind·ing
    habitual g.
    nonfunctional g.
    selective g.
    spot g.

grind·ing-in

Grip ce·ment

groove
 abutment g.
 alar g.
 alveolingual g.
 alveolobuccal g.
 alveololabial g.
 alveololingual g.
 buccal g.
 buccal developmental g.
 central g.
 central developmental g.
 dental g., primitive
 developmental g's
 distobuccal g.
 distobuccal developmental
  g.
 distolingual g.
 distolingual developmental
  g.
 enamel g's
 free gingival g.
 gingival g.
 inferior dental g.
 interdental g.
 lingual g.
 lingual developmental g.
 mesiobuccal g.
 mesiobuccal developmental
  g.
 mesiolingual g.
 mesiolingual
  developmental g.
 mylohyoid g.
 mylohyoid g. of inferior
  maxillary bone
 nasolabial g.
 nasomaxillary g.
 nasopalatine g.
 nasopharyngeal g.
 occlusal g.
 palatine g., anterior
 palatine g's of maxilla
 palatine g. of palatine bone
 palatomaxillary g.
 palatomaxillary g. of
  palatine bone
 pharyngeal g.
 pharyngotympanic g.

groove *(continued)*
 supplemental g's

groov·ing

growth
 condylar g.

Gru·ber
 Meckel-G. syndrome

G-type ream·er

guard
 bite g.
 mouth g.
 night g.
 occlusal g.

Gué·rin
 G's fracture

guid·ance
 condylar g.
 cuspid g.
 incisal g.

guide
 adjustable anterior g.
 anterior g.
 Bioform extended-range
  shade g.
 body porcelain shade g.
 condylar g.
 G. to Dental Materials and
  Devices
 drill g.
 incisal g.
 shade g.
 tooth shade g.

guide·line
 clasp g.
 health care g's

gum
 free g.

Gum-Aid paste

gun
 Messing g.
 root canal g.

Gun·ning
   G's splint

gut·ta-per·cha
   g.-p. baseplate
   g.-p. cone

gut·ta-per·cha *(continued)*
   g.-p. point
   SuccessFil g.-p.

Gy·si
   G's articulator

H

HA
 hydroxyapatite

Haas
 H. expansion appliance

HA coat·ed Mi·cro-Vent im·plant

HA coat·ed Screw-Vent im·plant

hab·it
 clamping h.
 clenching h.
 gnashing h.
 grinding h.
 masticatory h.
 oral h.
 tongue h.

Ha·bi·trol

ha·bit·u·al

Hade
 H.-Ring attachment

HAI
 hydroxyapatite-coated
  implant

Haj·du
 H.-Cheney syndrome

Hal·ci·on

Hall
 Pallister-H. syndrome

Hal·ler·mann
 H.-Streiff syndrome

hal·o·thane

Hal·sted
 H's mosquito hemostat

ham·mer
 dental h.

Ham·mond
 H's splint

Han·au
 H. articulators
 H. 130-21 articulator
 H. face-bows
 H's law of articulation

Hand
 H.-Schüller-Christian
  disease

Handi-Lin·er cav·i·ty lin·er

han·dle
 test h.
 Unigauge h.

hand·piece
 air-bearing turbine h.
 bayonet h.
 contra-angle h.
 Giromatic h.
 high-speed h's
 Racer h.
 right-angle h.
 straight h.
 ultra-high-speed h.
 ultrasonic h.
 water-turbine h.

Han·no·ver
 H's intermediate
  membrane

Haps·burg
 H. jaw
 H. lip

Hap·set hy·drox·y·ap·a·tite
 bone graft plas·ter

hard·en·ing
 age h.
 order-disorder h.
 precipitation h.
 strain h.
 work h.

hard·ness
 Brinell h. number (BHN)

hard·ness *(continued)*
    Brinell h. scale
    Brinell h. test
    diamond pyramid h.
    Knoop h. number (KHN)
    Knoop h. scale
    Knoop h. test
    material h.
    Mohs h. number (MHN)
    Mohs h. test
    h. number
    Rockwell h. number (RHN)
    Rockwell h. scale
    Rockwell h. test
    h. scale
    Vickers h. number (VHN)
    Vickers h. scale
    Vickers h. test

har·mo·ny
    occlusal h.
    occlusal h., functional

Hart
    H.-Dunn attachment

Har·vey chem·i·clave

Har·vold
    H. activator
    H. analysis
    H. standard values

Hatch
    H. clamp

hatch·et
    enamel h.

Haw·ley
    H. appliance
    H. bite plate
    H. retainer

Hay
    H.-Wells syndrome

HBO
    hyperbaric oxygen

head
    angular h. of quadratus
    labii superioris muscle

head *(continued)*
    h. of condyloid process of
    mandible
    infraorbital h. of quadratus
    labii superioris muscle
    little h. of mandible
    h. of mandible
    nasal h. of levator labii
    superioris alaeque nasi
    muscle
    zygomatic h. of quadratus
    labii superioris muscle

head·ache
    cluster h.

head·cap

head·gear
    cervical h.
    circumcranial orthodontic
    h.
    high-pull h.
    J-hook h.
    Kloehn-type h.
    orthodontic h.
    reverse-pull h.

heal·ing
    bone h.

heat·er
    compound h.

Heath
    H's operation

Heck
    H's disease

Hed·ström
    H. file

Heer·fordt
    H's syndrome

He·gar
    Olsen-H. needle holder

Heid·brink
    H. elevator
    H. root pick
    H. root-tip pick

height
  h. of contour
  h. of contour, surveyed
  cusp h.
  facial h.

He·lio·bond bond·ing agent

He·lio·mo·lar com·pos·ite res·in

He·lio·mo·lar res·in

He·lio·Pro·gress res·in

He·lio·seal pit and fis·sure seal·ant

He·lio·tint

he·lix
  quad h.

HEMA
  hydroxymethyl
    methacrylate

hem·an·gio·en·do·the·li·o·ma
  epithelioid h.

hem·an·gi·o·ma
  h. of bone
  central h.
  h. of jaw
  sclerosing h.

hem·a·to·ma *pl.* hem·a·tomas
  sublingual h.

hemi·fa·cial

hemi·glos·sec·to·my

hemi·man·dib·u·lec·to·my

hemi·max·il·lec·to·my

hemi·pal·ate

hemi·sec·to·my

He·mo·dent

he·mo·phil·ia

he·mor·rhage
  alveolar h.

he·mor·rhage *(continued)*
  gingival h.
  postextraction h.

he·mor·rha·gic

he·mo·stat
  Crile h.
  Halsted's mosquito h.
  Kelly h.
  Rochester-Péan h.

he·mo·stat·ic
  adsorbable h.

Hen·a·han
  H. periosteal elevator
  H. retractor

Henke-Ject sy·ringe

Hen·le
  external tuber of H.

hep·a·ran sul·fate

Herbst
  H. appliance

Her·cu·lite Con·dens·able com·pos·ite res·in

Her·cu·lite XR com·pos·ite ma·te·ri·al

Her·cu·lite XR gel etch·ant

Her·cu·lite XRV com·pos·ite res·in

he·red·i·tary

herp·an·gi·na

her·pes
  primary h. simplex
  recurrent intraoral h.
  recurrent h. labialis
  h. simplex
  type I vs. type II h.
  h. zoster

her·pet·i·form

Hert·wig
  H. sheath

Hert·wig *(continued)*
    sheath of H.

het·ero·dont

hexa·chlo·ro·phene

hexo·bar·bi·tal

H-Files

High·more
    antrum of H.

Hi·Lite bleach·ing sys·tem

hinge-bow

Hirsch·feld
    H's canal
    H. file
    H's silver point
    H.-Dunlop file

his·tio·cyte
    foamy h.
    phagocytic h.

his·tio·cy·to·ma
    atypical fibrous h.
    benign fibrous h.
    fibrous h.
    inflammatory fibrous h.
    malignant h.
    malignant fibrous h.

his·tio·cy·to·sis
    idiopathic h.
    h. X

His·to·plas·ma
    H. capsulatum

his·to·plas·mo·sis

Ho
    holmium

Hodg·kin
    H's disease
    Rapp-H. ectodermal
        dysplasia syndrome

hoe
    h. scaler
    surgical h.

Hold·away
    H. cephalometric
        standards

hold·er
    Baumgartner needle h.
    Boynton needle h.
    Castroviejo needle h.
    Collier needle h.
    Crile-Wood needle h.
    Derf needle h.
    foil h.
    Hegar-Baumgartner
        needle h.
    Mathieu needle h.
    matrix h.
    Mayo-Hegar needle h.
    needle h.
    Olsen-Hegar needle h.
    rubber dam h.
    Ryder needle h.

Hol·len·back
    H. carver
    H. condenser

Hol·lis·ter
    Levy-H. syndrome

hol·low
    Sebileau's h.

hol·mi·um

ho·mo·dont

hood
    tooth h.

hook
    bone h.
    elastic h.
    embrassure h.
    incisal h.
    intermaxillary h.
    labial h.
    molar h.
    sliding h.

Ho·ri·co Dia·flex dia·mond
    disk

Ho·ri·co Rib·bon Saw

hor·i·zon·tal
    Frankfort h.

horn
    h. of pulp

Hor·ner
    H. syndrome

Hors·ley
    H's wax

How
    H. crown pliers

Ho·ward
    H. apexo root pick
    H. file

How·med·i·ca dy·nam·ic com·pres·sion plate

Ho:YAG
    holmium:yttrium-aluminum-garnet

Ho:YAG (holmium:yttrium-aluminum-garnet) la·ser

Hru·ska
    H. attachment

HS-1 amal·ga·ma·tor

HTR poly·mer

HTR-MFI im·plant

H-type file

H-type root ca·nal file

Hue·ter
    Vogt-H. point

Hum·by
    H. knife

Hun·suck
    H. sagittal split osteotomy

Hunt·er
    bands of H.-Schreger
    H's syndrome

Hur·ler
    H's syndrome

Hur·ler *(continued)*
    H.-Scheie compound syndrome

Hur·ri·caine

hy·al·uro·nate

Hy-Bond ce·ment

Hy-Bond poly·car·box·yl·ate ce·ment

Hy-Bond Zinc Ox·ide Eu·gen·ol Tem·po·rary Ce·ment

Hy-Bond Zinc Phos·phate Ce·ment

hy·brid
    Z100 restorative spherical h.

Hy·dent den·ture in·di·ca·tor paste

Hy·dro·cal den·tal stone

Hy·dro-Cast den·ture re·lin·er

hy·dro·co·done bi·tar·trate

hy·dro·col·loid
    irreversible h.
    reversible h.
    SuperBody h.
    Versatile h.

Hy·dro·cryl den·ture re·line

Hy·dro-Jel Al·gi·nate

Hy·dro·plas·tic bor·der mold·ing ma·te·ri·al

Hy·dro·plas·tic tray ma·te·ri·al

Hy·dro·sil im·pres·sion ma·te·ri·al

Hy·dro·sil XT im·pres·sion ma·te·ri·al

hy·droxy·ap·a·tite
    nonporous h.

hy·droxy·ap·a·tite *(continued)*
    OsteoGen low temperature
       h.

hy·droxy·eth·yl meth·ac·ry·
    late

hy·drox·yl·ap·a·tite

Hy·drox·y·line cav·i·ty lin·er

hy·giene
    dental h.
    mouth h.
    oral h.

hy·gien·ist
    dental h.
    Registered Dental H.
       (RDH)

hy·gro·ma *pl.* hy·gro·mas, hy·
    gro·ma·ta
    cystic h.

hy·per·ce·men·to·sis

hy·per·don·tia

hy·per·ker·a·to·sis

hy·per·para·thy·roid·ism

hy·per·pla·sia
    adenomatoid h.
    cementum h.
    condylar h.
    coronoid h.
    Dilantin h.
    drug-induced gingival h.
    follicular lymphoid h.
       (FLH)
    gingival h.
    inflammatory papillary h.
    lymphoid h.
    mandibular h.
    maxillary h.
    palatal papillary h.
    papillary h.

hy·per·pla·sia *(continued)*
    pseudoepitheliomatous h.
    sebaceous h.
    verrucous h.

hy·per·plas·tic

hy·per·tau·ro·don·tism

hy·per·ther·mia
    malignant h.

hy·per·thy·roid·ism

hy·per·tro·phy
    hemifacial h.
    hemimandibular h.

Hy·po-Cal cal·ci·um hy·drox·
    ide paste

Hypo-Cal paste

hy·po·cone

hy·po·con·id

hy·po·con·u·lid

hy·po·don·tia

hy·po·glos·sal

hy·pog·na·thous

hy·po·mo·bil·i·ty
    mandibular h.

hy·po·para·thy·roid·ism

hy·po·phos·pha·ta·sia

hy·po·pla·sia
    condylar h.
    enamel h.
    malar h.
    mandibular h.
    maxillary h.
    midface h.

hy·po·thy·roid·ism

hy·pox·ia
    diffusion h.

hyp·si·sta·phyl·ia

IADR
  International Association for Dental Research

IAG
  International Academy of Gnathology

IAO
  International Association for Orthodontics

IAOM
  International Association of Oral Myology

I bar

id·io·path·ic

Im·age al·loy

im·mo·bil·iza·tion
  mandibular i.
  tooth i.

im·mo·bi·lize

IMNN
  isolated, nontraumatic mental branch neuropathy

im·pac·tion
  dental i.
  distoangular i.
  food i.
  food i., lateral
  horizontal i.
  mesioangular i.
  vertical i.

im·pac·tions

Im·per·va Bond den·tin prim·er

Im·per·va Du·al ad·he·sive res·in

im·pe·ti·go

im·pinge·ment

Im·pla·care cu·rette

im·plant
  abutment i.
  alloplastic i.
  alloplastic mesh i.
  alumina ceramic i.
  i. anchor
  anterior subperiosteal i.
  Apaceram i.
  Bio-Vent i.
  blade i's
  Brnemark I. System
  i. button
  ceramic endosseous i.
  CM endosseous i.
  collagen-hydroxyapatite i's
  complete subperiosteal i.
  composite allogeneic bone/alloplastic i's
  condylar i's
  Core-Vent i's
  cosmetic i's
  dental i's
  i. denture
  endodontic i.
  endodontic endosseous i.
  endosseous i's
  endosseous vent i.
  endosteal i.
  endosteal osseointegrated i's
  fabricated i.
  i. framework
  glenoid fossa i's
  gold dental i's
  HA-coated i.
  HA coated Micro-Vent i.
  HA coated Screw-Vent i.
  helicoid endosseus i.
  hexed cylinder i.
  HL antirotation i.
  HTR-MFI i.

im·plant *(continued)*
hydroxyapatite-bone i's
hydroxyapatite-coated i.
(HAI)
Integral i.
Integral Omniloc i.
intermediate i. structure
Interpore i's
intraosseous i.
intraperiosteal i.
magnet i.
magnetic i.
i. mesostructure
Micro-Vent dental i.
i. model
monostructure i.
mucosal i.
i. neck
needle endosseous i.
Nobelpharma endosseous
i's
Omniloc i.
oral i's
Osseodent i.
osseointegrated i.
OsteoGen i.
pin endosseous i.
polylactide osteosynthesis
i's
polymer tooth i.
polysulfone i's
porous hydroxyapatite i's
Proplast-Teflon TMJ i.
RA-2 ramus frame i's
i. restoration
i. screw
screw-type i's
Screw-Vent i.
self-tapping i.
Silastic i.
silicone rubber i's
Spectra-System dental i.
spiral endosseous i.
Steri-Oss i.
stock i.
subdermal i.
subperiosteal i.

im·plant *(continued)*
subperiosteal i. one-phase
technique
i. substructure
i. substructure interspace
i. superstructure neck
Swede-Vent dental i.
TCP i's
temporary i.
superstructure
titanium i.
transmandibular i's
transosseous i.
transosteal i.
Tubinger i.
two-piece i.
unilateral subperiosteal i.
universal subperiosteal i.
zygomatic i's

im·plan·ta·tion

im·plan·to·don·tics

im·plan·to·don·tist

im·plan·to·don·tol·o·gy

im·plan·tol·o·gist

im·plan·tol·o·gy
dental i.
oral i.

Im·pre·gum F im·pres·sion ma
·te·ri·al

im·pres·sion
im·pres·sion
alginate i's
anatomic i.
basilar i.
bridge i.
cleft palate i.
closed mouth i.
complete denture i.
composite i.
i. compound
correctable i.
corrective i.
dental i.

im·pres·sion *(continued)*
    digastric i.
    direct i.
    direct bone i.
    elastic i.
    final i.
    fluid wax i.
    functional i.
    hydrocolloid i. (reversible and irreversible)
    Jeltrate alginate i's
    lower i.
    mandibular i.
    i. material
    maxillary i.
    modeling plastic i.
    partial denture i.
    pickup i.
    pickup i., subperiosteal
    i. plaster
    plaster i.
    preliminary i.
    prepared cavity i.
    presurgical i.
    primary i.
    secondary i.
    sectional i.
    silicone i.
    snap i.
    subperiosteal pickup i.
    surgical bone i.
    Thiokol rubber i.
    trigeminal i. of temporal bone
    upper i.
    wash i.
    i. wax
    wax i.
    welded inlay i.

Im·print im·pres·sion ma·te·ri·al

IMZ Hex Im·plant Sys·tem

In-Ce·ram

in·ci·sal

in·ci·sion
    angular i.

in·ci·sion *(continued)*
    bicoronal i.
    Blair i.
    butterfly i.
    external bevel i.
    Fergusson's i.
    hemicoronal i.
    inner bevel i.
    internal bevel i.
    inverse bevel i.
    inverted bevel i.
    marginal i.
    preauricular i.
    relieving i.
    retromandibular i.
    reverse bevel i.
    Risdon i.
    trapezoid i.
    Weber-Fergusson i.
    Wilde's i.

in·ci·sive

in·ci·so·la·bi·al

in·ci·so·lin·gual

in·ci·so·prox·i·mal

in·ci·sor
    central i.
    first i.
    hawk-bill i's
    lateral i.
    medial i.
    second i.
    shovel-shaped i's
    winged i.

in·ci·sure
    i. of mandible
    semilunar i. of mandible
    sigmoid i. of mandible

in·cli·na·tion
    axial i.
    condylar guidance i.
    condylar guide i.
    lateral condylar i.
    lingual i.

in·cline
    distal i's
    guiding i's
    inner i's
    mesial i's
    outer i's

in·clu·sion
    dental i.

in·com·pe·tence
    lip i.
    oral i.

in·dent·er
    Brinell i.
    Knoop i.
    Rockwell i.
    Vickers i.

in·dex *pl.* in·dex·es, in·di·ces
    alveolar i.
    auricular i.
    auriculoparietal i.
    cephalic i.
    cephalo-orbital i.
    debris i.
    dental i.
    I. to Dental Literature
    Dunning-Leach i.
    facial i.
    Flower's i.
    Gingival I.
    gingival i. (GI)
    gingival-bone i.
    gingival-bone count i.
    gingival periodontal i.
    gingival recession i.
    gnathic i.
    Greene-Vermillion i.
    height i.
    height-breadth i.
    height-length i.
    irritation i.
    Löe i.
    maxilloalveolar i.
    Mohs i.
    morphologic face i.
    oral hygiene i.
    palatal i.

in·dex *(continued)*
    palatal height i.
    palatine i.
    palatomaxillary i.
    periodontal i.
    periodontal disease i.
    physiognomic upper face i.
    plaque i. (PI)
    PMA (papilla, gingival
        margin, and attached
        gingiva) i.
    Pont's i.
    Ramfjord i.
    i. of refraction
    refraction i.
    retention i.
    Russell i.
    simplified calculus i. (CI-S)
    simplified debris i. (DI-S)
    simplified oral hygiene i.
        (OHI-S)
    therapeutic i.
    vertical i.

in·di·ca·tor
    Attest biological i's
    Tooth Color I.

In·dic Die Stone den·tal stone

in·fec·tion
    apical i.
    bone necrosis and i.
    cervicofacial i's
    Plaut-Vincent i.
    periodontal i.
    Vincent's i.

in·fec·tious

in·flam·ma·to·ry

in·fra·bulge

in·fra·clu·sion

in·fra·den·ta·le

in·fra·man·dib·u·lar

in·fra·max·il·lary

in·fra·struc·ture
    implant i.

in·fra·ver·sion

In·gras·sia
    apophysis of I.

in·jec·tion
    epinephrine i.
    intrapulpal i.
    intraseptal i.

in·jury
    avulsion i.
    dentoalveolar i.

in·lay
    American Gold "M-H" i.
    American Gold "M" i.
     medium
    Baker i.
    Baker i., extra hard
    Baker i., hard
    i. burnout
    cast i.
    i. casting wax
    Crown K i.
    epithelial i.
    gold i.
    Goldsmith I i.
    i. II B
    Jelenko special i.
    Leff light i.
    Libra II i. and crown
    Mowrey B i.
    i. pattern wax
    porcelain i.
    Sterngold i.
    Sterngold Bridgette i.
    Veribest 22 Kt i.

in·sert
    intramucosal i.
    mucosal i.

in·ser·tion

In·sta-Glaze pol·ish·ing paste

in·stru·ment
    beam guiding i.

in·stru·ment *(continued)*
    carving i.
    cavity i.
    composite filling i's
    condensing i.
    cone-socket i.
    contouring i.
    cutting i.
    dental i.
    diamond rotary i.
    double-ended i.
    endodontic i.
    filling i.
    i. grasp
    Gregg filling i.
    hand i.
    handcutting i.
    Kirkland i's
    long-handled i.
    McCain i's
    occlusal adjustment i's
    orthodontic i.
    P.K. Thomas waxing i.
    paralleling i.
    periodontal i.
    root canal i.
    root canal therapy i.
    rotary i.
    ultrasonic i's
    Wall waxing i.
    waxing i.
    Woodson filling i.

in·stru·men·tal

in·stru·men·tar·i·um

in·stru·men·ta·tion

In·sure res·in ce·ment

in·ta·glio

In·te·gral im·plant

In·te·gral Om·ni·loc im·plant

in·ter·al·ve·o·lar

in·ter·cus·pal

in·ter·cus·pa·tion

in·ter·cusp·ing

in·ter·dent

in·ter·den·tal

in·ter·den·ta·le

in·ter·den·ti·um

in·ter·dig·i·ta·tion

in·ter·face
    bone i.

In·ter·face cav·i·ty lin·er

in·ter·fer·ence
    cuspal i.
    occlusal i's

in·ter·fur·ca *pl.* in·ter·fur·cae

in·ter·fur·cae

in·ter·go·ni·al

in·ter·max·il·lary

in·ter·nal

In·ter·na·tion·al Acad·e·my of
    Gnath·ol·o·gy

In·ter·na·tion·al As·so·ci·a·
    tion for Den·tal Re·search

In·ter·na·tion·al As·so·ci·a·
    tion of Oral My·ol·o·gy

In·ter·na·tion·al As·so·ci·a·
    tion for Or·tho·don·tics

In·ter·na·tion·al Col·lege of
    Den·tists

in·ter·oc·clu·sal

In·ter·pore 200

In·ter·pore Hex Im·plant Sys·
    tem

In·ter·pore im·plants

in·ter·prox·i·mal

In·ter·val ce·ment

In·ter·val fill·ing ma·te·ri·al

in·tra·bony

in·tra·buc·cal

in·tra·ep·i·the·li·al

in·tra·mu·co·sal

in·tra·oral

in·tra·os·se·ous

in·tra·ver·sion

in·tro·ver·sion

in·tru·sion

in·tu·ba·tion
    nasotracheal i.
    orotracheal i.

in·va·gi·na·tus

in·vest

in·vest·ing
    i. the pattern
    vacuum i.

in·vest·ment
    cast i.
    cristobalite i.
    dental i.
    quartz i.
    refractory i.

ion·o·mer
    EMKA-Fil glass i.
    glass i.
    VariGlass glass i.

Ion·os·cem ce·ment

Ion·o·sphere al·loy

ion·to·pho·re·sis
    fluoride i.

IPC in·ter·prox·i·mal carv·er

ipro·pla·tin

Ip·so·clip at·tach·ment

Iris
    I. scissors

IRM re·stor·a·tive

ir·ri·ga·tion
    endodontic i.
    oral i.

ir·ri·ga·tor
    Max-I-Probe i.
    oral i.

ir·ri·ta·bil·i·ty

ir·ri·ta·tion

Iso·caine

iso·eth·a·rine

iso·flu·rane

Iso·lit Wax Re·lease Agent

iso·pro·pyl pal·mi·tate

iso·pro·te·re·nol

iter
    i. dentium

ITI Den·tal Im·plant Sys·tem

ITI non-sub·merged den·tal
    im·plant sys·tem

itra·con·a·zole

ivo·ry

Ivory clamp

Ivory for·ceps

Ivory rub·ber dam clamp for·
    ceps

IVRO
    intraoral vertical ramus
      osteotomy

Ivy
    I. loop
    I. loop wiring

jack·et
  porcelain j.

jack·screw
  j. appliance
  j. regainer-maintainer

Jack·son
  J's appliance
  J. crib

Jac·quart
  J's angle

Jam·pel
  Schwartz-J. syndrome

Ja·pan wax

Ja·quette
  J. scaler

Ja·ra·bak
  J. pliers

jaun·dice

jaw
  bird-beak j.
  j. brace
  crackling j.
  Hapsburg j.
  lower j.
  parrot j.
  pipe j.
  upper j.

JD al·loy

Jef·fer·son
  J. fracture

Jeg·hers
  Peutz-J. syndrome

Jel·cone im·pres·sion ma·te·ri·al

Je·len·ko Dur·o·cast

Je·len·ko Mod·u·lay

Je·len·ko No. 7 gold al·loy

Je·len·ko spe·cial in·lay

Je·len·ko su·per wire

Je·len·ko sur·vey·or

Jel-Span al·loy

Jel-Thin 9 disk

Jel·trate al·gi·nate im·pres·sions

Jel·trate im·pres·sion ma·te·ri·al

Jel·trate Plus im·pres·sion ma·te·ri·al

Jen·kins
  J. porcelain

Job
  J's syndrome

Jo·han·son
  J.-Blizzard syndrome

Joh·ni·chi
  J. torque gauge

John·son
  J. method
  J. pliers
  J. twin wire appliance
  Stevens-J. syndrome

John·ston
  J.-Callahan diffusion technique

joint
  Ackermann bar j.
  atlantoaxial j.
  atlanto-occipital j.
  bar j.
  single sleeve bar j.
  Steiger's j.
  temporomandibular j.

Jones
  J. nasal splint

Jones *(continued)*
    J. 1 test
    J. 2 test

Jor·gen·sen
    J. technique

Jo·seph
    J's clamp
    J's saw

jump·ing
    j. the bite

junc·tion
    alar-facial j.
    amelodentinal j.
    cementodentinal j.
    cementoenamel j.
    dentin-cementum j.
    dentin-enamel j.

junc·tion *(continued)*
    dentinocemental j.
    dentinoenamel j.
    dentogingival j.
    dermoepidermal j.
    intermediate j.
    interneuronal j. j.
    mucogingival j.
    myoneural j.
    osseous j's
    synaptic j.
    tight j.

junc·tion·al

jur·is·pru·dence
    dental j.

Jus·ti res·in ce·ment

Just Treat·ment re·lin·er

Ka·don cav·i·ty lin·er

Ka·don res·in fill·ing ma·te·ri·al

Kai·ser
Kirkland-K. pack

Kal·gi·nate im·pres·sion ma·te·ri·al

K4 an·chor sys·tem

Kap·lan
Crane K. scaler

Ka·po·si
K's sarcoma

Ka·rid·i·um li·quid

Ka·rid·i·um phos·phate flu·o·ride top·i·cal gel

Ka·rol·yi
K. effect

Ka·zan·jian
K. forceps
K's operation
K's splint
K. T bar

Keil
K. bone

Kel·ly
K. hemostat
K. scissors

ke·loid
k. of gums

Ken·a·log 40

Ken·ne·dy
K. bar
K. classification (for partially edentulous arches)

Kent zinc ce·ment

ker·a·tin·iza·tion

ker·a·to·ac·an·tho·ma

ker·a·to·cyst
odontogenic k's

ker·a·top·a·thy
band k.

ker·a·to·sis *pl.* ker·a·to·ses
actinic k.
seborrheic k.

Kerr com·pos·ite fin·ish·ing sys·tem

Kerr En·do·post Sys·tem

Kerr equal·iz·ing paste

Kerr file

Kerr hard wax

Kerr Lur·a·lite

Kerr Perm·plas·tic

Kerr ream·er

Kerr reg·u·lar wax

Kerr seal·er

Kerr Spe·ra·loy

Kerr Spher-A-Caps

Kerr Top·i·cal Flu·ra-Gel

Kerr Tray·con

Kes·ling
K. appliance
K. spring

Ke·tac-Bond Ap·li·cap ce·ment

Ke·tac-Bond ce·ment

Ke·tac-Cem Ap·li·cap ce·ment

Ke·tac-Cem MAXI·CAP ce·ment

Ke·tac-Cem ra·dio·paque ce·ment

Ke·tac-Fil re·stor·a·tive

Ke·tac glass-ion·o·mer seal·er

Ke·tac-Glaze

Ke·tac-Sil·ver glass ion·o·mer/
sil·ver re·stor·a·tive

ke·ta·mine

ke·to·con·a·zole

key
    dental k.
    screw post k.
    torquing k.

Key-To al·gi·nate im·pres·sion
  ma·te·ri·al

key·way

K-Files

K-Flex files

KHN
    Knoop hardness number

Kil·li·an
    K. and Teschler-Nicola
      syndrome

Kings·ley
    K. appliance
    K. plate
    K. splint

Kirk·land
    K. chisel
    K. curet
    K. instrument
    K. knife
    K. periodontal pack
    K. scaler
    K.-Kaiser pack

Kirsch·ner
    K. pins
    K. wire

kit
    Messerann k.

Klammt
    K. activator

Kleb·si·el·la

Klip·pel
    K.-Feil deformity
    K.-Feil sequence

Kloehn
    K.-type headgear

Kniest
    K's disease

knife
    Blair k.
    Buck k.
    button k.
    carving k.
    cautery k.
    electric k.
    endotherm k.
    finishing k.
    gingivectomy k.
    gold k.
    Goldman-Fox k.
    Goldman-Fox spear k.
    Humby k.
    interdental k.
    Kirkland k.
    Merrifield's k.
    Monahan-Lewis k.
    Orban k.
    periodontal k.
    plaster k.

Knoop
    K. hardness
    K. hardness indenter point
    K. hardness number
    K. indenter
    K. indenter point
    K. scale

knot
    enamel k.

Koch·er
    K's operation

Koeb·er
    K's saw

Kole
    K. procedure

Koo·lin·er den·ture re·line

Korff
    K's fiber

ko·ro·ni·on *pl.* ko·ro·nia

Ko-type ream·er

Kri·mer
    K's operation

Krueg·er
    K. stop

K-type ream·er

K-type root ca·nal file

Ku·rer an·chor sys·tem

Kwik-Trays

K-wire

L
lambda
left

La
lambda

lab

La·bet·a·lol

la·bi·al·is

la·bio·al·ve·o·lar

la·bio·ax·io·gin·gi·val

la·bio·cer·vi·cal

la·bio·cli·na·tion

la·bio·den·tal

la·bio·gin·gi·val

la·bio·in·ci·sal

la·bio·lin·gual

la·bio·pal·a·tine

la·bio·place·ment

la·bio·plas·ty

la·bio·te·nac·u·lum

la·bio·ver·sion

la·bi·um *pl.* la·bia
l. mandibulare
l. maxillare

La·borde
L's forceps

la·bra·le

la·brum *pl.* la ·bra

Lab Stone den·tal stone

lac·to·fer·rin
salivary l.

La·da·more
L. plugger

La·grange
L's scissors

lamb·da

la·mel·la *pl.* la·mel·lae
enamel lamellae

lam·i·na *pl.* lam·i·nae
basal l.
basement l.
l. dura
palatine l. of maxilla

lam·i·nate
porcelain l.

lam·in·in

lamp
annealing l.
mouth l.

La·my
Maroteaux-L.
mucopolysaccharidosis
syndrome

lan·cet
gingival l.
gum l.

land·mark
craniometric l's

Lane
L. cleft palate needle
L's plate

Lan·gen·beck
L's pedicle mucoperiosteal
flap

Lan·ger
L. mesomelic dysplasia
L.-Giedion syndrome

lan·i·ary

Lar·sen
    L's syndrome

Lars·son
    Sjögren-L. syndrome

la·ser
    argon l.
    carbon dioxide l.
    Ho:YAG l.
    holmium:YAG l.
    holmium:yttrium-
        aluminum-garnet
        (Ho:YAG) l.
    Nd:YAG l.
    neodymium:YAG l.
    neodymium:yttrium-
        aluminum-garnet
        (Nd:YAG) l.
    TwoPointOne XE l.

Las·sar
    L's paste

lat·er·al

lathe
    dental laboratory l.

lat·tice
    Brevais l.
    crystal l.
    cubic l.
    hexagonal l.
    l. imperfection
    orthorhombic l.
    space l.

law
    l's of articulation
    Hanau's l's of articulation

Lax·o·va
    Neu-L. syndrome

lay·er
    adamantine l.
    ameloblastic l.
    aponeurosis l.
    enamel l., inner
    enamel l., outer
    granular l. of Tomes

lay·er *(continued)*
    odontoblastic l.
    submantle l.
    subodontoblastic l.
    Tomes' granular l.
    Weil's basal l.

LE
    lupus erythematosus

Leach
    Dunning-L. index

ledge
    crown l.

ledg·ing

Lee
    L. denture

Le·fevre
    Papillon-L. syndrome

Leff
    L. light inlay

Le Fort
    Le F. fracture
    Le F. osteotomy
    Le F. I downfracture
    Le F. I downfracture
        osteotomy
    Le F. I osteotomy
    Le F. I maxillary
        advancement
    Le F. I maxillary
        osteotomy
    Le F. III fracture
    Le F. III midface
        advancement
    Le F. III osteotomy

Le·gan
    L. and Burstone
        cephalometric standards

leio·myo·ma
    vascular l.

leio·myo·sar·co·ma

Lem·li
    Smith-L.-Opitz syndrome

length
  arch l.
  basialveolar l.
  basinasal l.
  l. of crown, buccal
  l. of crown, labial
  dental l.
  gauge l.
  l. of mandible
  maxilloalveolar l.
  l. of palate
  l. of root
  span l.

len·ti·go *pl.* len·ti·gi·nes
  actinic l.
  l. simplex

len·tu·la

len·tu·lo

Lenz
  L.-Majewski hyperostosis
    syndrome

lep·ro·sy

lep·to·don·tous

lep·to·staph·y·line

Le·roy
  L. I-cell syndrome

le·sion
  benign fibro-osseous l.
  benign lymphoepithelial l.
  benign lymphoepithelial l.
    (BLEL) of salivary glands
  giant cell l's of the jaws
  kissing l.
  nasomaxillary giant cell l.

le·thal

leu·ke·mia
  acute myelogenous l.
  acute nonlymphocytic l.
    (ANLL)
  Burkitt's cell acute l.
  chronic myelogenous l.
    (CML)

leu·ko·ede·ma

leu·ko·pla·kia
  hairy l.
  proliferative verrucous l.

Le Vasseur
  Le V.-Merrill retractor

lev·el·ing

Le·vo·nor·def·rin

Le·vy
  L.-Hollister syndrome

Lew·is
  Monahan-L. knife

L for·ceps

LG al·loy

Lib·er·ty al·loy

Li·bra II in·lay and crown

Li·bra III crown and bridge

Lib·ri·um

li·chen
  l. planus

lick·ing
  lip l.

li·do·caine
  l. hydrochloride

Life pulp cap·ping ma·te·ri·al

lig·a·ment
  accessory l.
  accessory l. of Henle,
    lateral
  accessory l. of Henle,
    medial
  alar l's
  alveolodental l.
  apical dental l.
  apical odontoid l.
  arytenoepiglottic l.
  l's of auricle of external ear
  Berry's l.
  canthal l's

lig·a·ment *(continued)*
    capsular l's
    cemental l.
    ceratocricoid l.
    cricoarytenoid l., posterior
    cricopharyngeal l.
    cricosantorinian l.
    cricothyroarytenoid l.
    cricothyroid l.
    cricotracheal l.
    dental l.
    external l. of mandibular
      articulation
    Ferrein's l.
    gingivodental l.
    glenoid l. of mandibular
      fossa
    hammock l.
    Henle's l.
    hyoepiglottic l.
    interarticular l.
    intermaxillary l.
    lateral l. of
      temporomandibular
      articulation
    lateral l. of
      temporomandibular joint,
      external
    lateral l. of
      temporomandibular joint,
      internal
    Lockwood's suspensory l.
    maxillary l.
    maxillary l., lateral
    maxillary l., middle
    medial l. of
      temporomandibular
      articulation
    palpebral l., lateral
    palpebral l., medial
    periodontal l.
    petrosphenoid l.
    petrosphenoid l., anterior
    pharyngeal l.
    pterygomandibular l.
    pterygomaxillary l.
    pterygospinal l.
    salpingopharyngeal l.

lig·a·ment *(continued)*
    Sappey's l.
    sphenomandibular l.
    stylohyoid l.
    stylomandibular l.
    stylomaxillary l.
    stylomylohyoid l.
    suspensory l.
    sutural l.
    synovial l.
    temporomandibular l.
    thyroepiglottic l.
    thyrohyoid l.
    thyrohyoid l., median
    tracheal l's
    triquetral l.
    tubopharyngeal l. of
      Rauber
    l's of Valsalva
    ventricular l. of larynx
    vestibular l.
    vocal l.

lig·a·men·tum *pl.* lig·a·men·ta
    ligamenta alaria
    ligamenta annularia
      tracheae
    l. apicis dentis axis
    l. apicis dentis epistrophei
    ligamenta auricularia
    l. ceratocricoideum
    l. cricoarytenoideum
      posterius
    l. cricopharyngeum
    l. cricothyroideum
      medianum
    l. cricotracheale
    l. hyoepiglotticum
    l. hyothyreoideum laterale
    l. hyothyreoideum medium
    l. laterale articulationis
      temporomandibularis
    l. palpebrale laterale
    l. palpebrale mediale
    l. pterygospinale
    l. pterygospinosum
    l. sphenomandibulare
    l. stylohyoideum

lig·a·men·tum *(continued)*
    l. stylomandibulare
    l. temporomandibulare
    l. thyreoepiglotticum
    l. thyroepiglotticum
    l. thyrohyoideum laterale
    l. thyrohyoideum
      medianum
    l. ventriculare
    l. vestibulare
    l. vocale

li·ga·tion
    interdental l.
    tooth l.

lig·a·ture
    circummandibular l's
    grass-line l.
    steel l.
    suspension l's
    thread-elastic l.

lim·bus *pl.*lim·bi
    alveolar l. of mandible
    alveolar l. of maxilla
    l. alveolaris mandibulae
    l. alveolaris maxillae

Linc al·loy

Linde·mann
    L. bur

line
    accretion l's
    alveolobasilar l.
    auriculobregmatic l.
    basinasal l.
    basiobregmatic l.
    basion-nasion l.
    bismuth l.
    blue l.
    calcification l's
    cementing l's
    cervical l.
    contour l's
    copper l.
    Corrigan's l.
    Czermak's l's
    demarcation l.

line *(continued)*
    developmental l's
    l. of draw
    l's of Ebner
    facial l.
    finish l.
    Frankfort Horizontal l.
    fulcrum l.
    fulcrum l., retentive
    fulcrum l., stabilizing
    gingival l.
    gum l.
    high lip l.
    imbrication l's of
      cementum
    imbrication l's of Ebner
    imbrication l's of Pickerill
    incremental l's
    incremental l's of
      cementum
    incremental l's of Ebner
    lead l.
    lip l.
    lip l., high
    lip l., low
    load l.
    low lip l.
    mesenteric l.
    mucogingival l.
    mylohyoid l. of mandible
    mylohyoidean l.
    nasobasal l.
    nasobasilar l.
    neonatal l.
    oblique l. of mandible
    oblique l. of mandible,
      internal
    l. of occlusion
    l's of Owen
    Pickerill's imbrication l's
    Poirier's l.
    precentral l.
    recessional l's
    resorption l.
    resting l.
    retentive fulcrum l.
    Retzius' l's
    reversal l.

line *(continued)*
　　Salter's l's
　　l's of Schreger
　　segmental l's
　　stabilizing fulcrum l.
　　survey l.
　　Topinard's l.
　　Virchow's l.

lin·ea *pl.* lin·eae
　　l. alba

lin·er
　　BaseLine glass ionomer
　　　base/l.
　　Cavalite cavity l.
　　Cavitec cavity l.
　　cavity l.
　　Coe Rect denture l.
　　Coe-soft denture l.
　　cushion l.
　　Handi-L.
　　Handi-Liner cavity l.
　　Hydroxyline cavity l.
　　Interface cavity l.
　　Kadon cavity l.
　　Preline base/l.
　　resilient l.
　　soft l.
　　Speed l.
　　Timeline base/l.
　　Visco-gel tissue conditioner
　　　and l.
　　Vitrebond base/l.

lin·gual

lin·gua·le

lin·gu·la *pl.* lin·gu·lae
　　l. of lower jaw

lin·guo·ax·i·al

lin·guo·ax·io·gin·gi·val

lin·guo·cer·vi·cal

lin·guo·cli·na·tion

lin·guo·clu·sion

lin·guo·den·tal

lin·guo·dis·tal

lin·guo·gin·gi·val

lin·guo·in·ci·sal

lin·guo·me·si·al

lin·guo-oc·clu·sal

lin·guo·place·ment

lin·guo·pul·pal

lin·guo·ver·sion

lin·ing
　　cavity l.

lip
　　l. adhesion
　　cleft l.
　　double l.
　　Hapsburg l.
　　inferior l.
　　lower l.
　　superior l.
　　upper l.

li·pec·to·my
　　facial l.
　　submental l.

lip·id

lip·oid

li·po·ma
　　sublingual l.

lipo·sar·co·ma

Li·qua-Mark

liq·uid
　　Fluorident l.
　　Karidium l.
　　Nebs analgesic l.
　　Pulpdent l.
　　Topicale l.

li·sin·o·pril

Lis·ter
　　L. scissors

Lis·ter·ine

Lis·ton
    L's forceps
    L's operation
    L's scissors

Lite·Line den·tal re·line

Lit·tau·er
    L. scissors

Li·zars
    L. operation

load
    occlusal l.

lobe

lo·ca·tor
    abutment l.
    electronic apex l's

Lock·wood
    L's suspensory ligament

Löe
    L. index system

Lo·gan
    L. bow

Lo·ma Lin·da man·drel

loop
    alignment l.
    bite wing l's
    boot l.
    box l.
    cervical l.
    closing l.
    delta l.
    drag l.
    Ivy l.
    retraction l.
    segmental closing l.
    segmental retraction l.
    vertical l.
    wire l.

lor·a·ze·pam

Lor·cet 10/650

Lor·tab

loss
    edentulous bone l.

Lowe
    L. syndrome

Löw·en·berg
    L's forceps

Low·ry
    Coffin-L. syndrome

loz·enge
    benzocaine l's

LP-2 im·pres·sion ma·te·ri·al

Luc
    Caldwell-L. operation
    L's operation

Lu·cas
    L. curet

Lu·cite

Lu·ci·tone

Lu·ci·tone 199 den·ture base res·in

Lud·wig
    L's angina

Lueb·ke
    L.-Ochsenbein flap

Luer:Lok sy·ringe

lug
    retention l.

Luhr mi·cro·fix·a·tion sys·tem

lu·pus
    chronic cutaneous l.
     erythematosus
    discoid l.
    discoid l. erythematosus
     (DLE)
    l. erythematosus (LE)
    subacute l. erythematosus
     (SCLE)
    systemic l. erythematosus

Lur·a·lite im·pres·sion paste

Lur·ide drop

Lur·ide Lozi-Tabs

Lur·ide-SF Lozi-Tabs

Lur·ide top·i·cal gel

Lux·al·loy al·loy

Lux·al·loy amal·gam al·loy

Ly·ell
    L's disease

lym·phan·gi·o·ma

lym·pho·epi·the·li·al

lym·phoid

lym·pho·ma
    Burkitt's l.
    malignant l.
    non-Hodgkin's l's
    primary l. of bone

lym·pho·nod·u·lar

Ly·nal tis·sue con·di·tion·er

ly·so·zyme
    salivary l.

Mc·Cain
    M. bipolar cautery
    M. instruments
    M. monopolar cautery

Mc·Call
    M. curet
    M's festoon
    M. scaler

Mc·Col·lum
    M. attachment

Mc·Ew·en
    M's point

ma·chine
    casting m.
    Taggard's compressed-gas
        casting m.

Mc·Kel·lop
    M. pliers

mac·ro·don·tia

mac·ro·gen·ia

mac·ro·gin·gi·vae

mac·ro·glos·sia

mac·ro·gna·thia

mac·ro·sto·mia

mac·ro·tooth *pl.* mac·ro·teeth

Mc·Shir·ley
    M's electromallet

mac·ule
    caf au lait m's
    melanotic m.

Ma·gi·cian bur

Ma·Gill
    M. forceps

Mag·nan
    M's movement

Mag·na·sil pro·phy·lax·is
    paste

mag·net
    denture m.

main·tain·er
    band and bar space m.
    band and crib space m.
    band and loop space m.
    broken stress space m.
    cantilever space m.
    crown and bar space m.
    crown and crib space m.
    fixed-removable space m.
    fixed space m.
    Gerber space m.
    Mayne space m.
    removable space m.
    space m.

Ma·jew·ski
    Lenz-M. hyperostosis
        syndrome

Ma·jor·i·ty al·loy

mal·align·ment

Ma·lar·Pack

Ma·las·sez
    M. rest

mal·erup·tion

mal·for·ma·tion
    arteriovenous m. (AVM)
    congenital arteriovenous
        m.

mal·let

mal·oc·clu·sion
    class I m.
    class II m.
    class III m.
    closed-bite m.
    deflective m.
    open-bite m.

mal·po·si·tion
  jaw m.

mal·turned

mam·e·lon

man·di·ble

man·dib·u·lar

man·dib·u·lec·to·my

man·dib·u·lo·plas·ty

man·dib·u·lot·o·my

man·drel
  disk m.
  endosseous implant needle
    m.
  Loma Linda m.
  Moore's m.
  Morgan's m.
  pop-on m.
  snap-on m.
  Sof-Lex Pop-On m.

man·dril

manu·dy·na·mom·e·ter

Mar·caine

Mar·che·sa·ni
  Weill-M. syndrome

Mar·fan
  M's syndrome

mar·gin
  alveolar m. of mandible
  alveolar m. of maxilla
  free gingival m.
  free gum m.
  gingival m.
  gum m.
  incisal m.
  porcelain-fused-to-metal
    (PFM) m's

mar·go pl. mar·gi·nes
  m. alveolaris

mark·er
  periodontal pocket m.

mark·er (continued)
  Richey condyle m.

mark·ing
  carbon m.

Ma·ro·teaux
  M.-Lamy
    mucopolysaccharidosis
    syndrome

Mar·quis
  M. probe

Mar·shall
  M. syndrome
  M.-Smith syndrome

mar·su·pi·al·iza·tion

Mar·tin
  M. carver

Mary·land bridge ad·he·sive

mask
  gingival m.

mas·sage
  gingival m.

Mas·son tri·chrome stain

Mas·ter Tray

mas·tic

mas·ti·ca·tion
  bilateral m.
  unilateral m.

mas·ti·ca·to·ry

mas·ti·che

ma·te·ria
  m. alba
  m. dentica

ma·te·ri·al
  Accoe impression m.
  Accoe tray M.
  Adaptol impression m.
  Adaptol thermoplastic
    impression m.
  agar impression m.

ma·te·ri·al *(continued)*
  Algident impression m.
  alginate impression m.
  Alkaliner calcium
    hydroxide m.
  baseplate m.
  Baysilex Hydroactiv
    impression m.
  Baysilex impression m.
  bite registration m.
  blockout m.
  Blue Core Build Up m.
  cast m.
  Cavit filling m.
  Cavit G temporary filling
  Cavit temporary filling m.
  Cavit W temporary filling
    m.
  chairside reline m.
  Cinch-Vinyl impression m.
  Citricon impression m.
  coating m.
  Coe-flex impression m.
  colloid impression m.
  composite m.
  core m.
  CutterJel impression m.
  CutterSil impression m.
  CutterSil Mucosa silicone
    impression m.
  CutterSil XL silocone
    impression m.
  Deelastic impression m.
  Deguflex Monophase
    polysiloxane impression
    m.
  dental m.
  duplicating m.
  elastic impression m.
  elastomeric impression m.
  EMKA-Silver core m.
  Exaflex impression m.
  Examix impression m.
  Express bite registration
    m.
  Express impression m.
  Extrude Extra impression
    m.

ma·te·ri·al *(continued)*
  Extrude impression m.
  m. fatigue
  filling m.
  Flexicon impression m.
  FluoroCore core m.
  Gore-Tex regenerative m.
  m. hardness
  heavy body impression m.
  Herculite XR composite m.
  hydrocolloid impression m.
  Hydroplastic border
    molding m.
  Hydroplastic tray m.
  Hydrosil impression m.
  Hydrosil XT impression m.
  Impregum F impression m.
  impression m.
  Imprint impression m.
  inelastic impression m.
  Interval filling m.
  investment m.
  irreversible hydrocolloid
    impression m.
  Jelcone impression m.
  Jeltrate impression m.
  Jeltrate Plus impression
    m.
  Kadon resin filling m.
  Kalginate impression m.
  Key-To alginate
    impression m.
  Life pulp capping m.
  light body impression m.
  Lite Line soft denture
    reline m.
  LP-2 impression m.
  Lynal soft liner m's
  Memosil m.
  Memosil bite registration
    m.
  Miracle Mix core m.
  Neo-Plex impression m.
  Omni Flex impression m.
  Opotow Jelset impression
    m.
  Oryl denture lining m.
  Palginex 75 impression m.

ma·te·ri·al *(continued)*
    Perfourm Hydroactiv
      impression m.
    Peripac periodontal
      packaging m.
    Permadyne Garant
      impression m.
    Permadyne impression m.
    Permagum Garant
      impression m.
    Permagum impression m.
    Permlastic impression m.
    plaster impression m.
    polyether impression m.
    Polyjel NF impression m.
    polysulfide impression m.
    Precise impression m.
    President impression m.
    ProFlex impression m.
    Pro-Temp crown and
      bridge m.
    provisionally acceptable m.
    Ramitec bite registration
      m.
    Recon tissue conditioner
      and functional
      impression m.
    refractory m.
    Regisil bite registration m.
    regular body impression m.
    reline m.
    Reprosil impression m.
    restorative m.
    reversible hydrocolloid
      impression m.
    rubber base impression m.
    rubber impression m.
    Rubberloid impression m.
    Silene silicone impression
      m.
    silicone impression m.
    SIR impression m.
    Snap crown and bridge m.
    Stat BR bite registration
      m.
    Softone tissue conditioner
      and functional
      impression m.

ma·te·ri·al *(continued)*
    Supergel impression m.
    Sta-Tic impression m.
    Super Rubber impression
      m.
    Supersil impression m.
    Surflex F impression m.
    Surgident impression m.
    Tempit filling and seal m.
    temporary m.
    thermoplastic impression
      m.
    Ti-Core core m.
    tissue equivalent m.
    Triad provisional m.
    Triad VLC direct reline m.
    unacceptable m.
    UniJel impression m.
    vinyl polysiloxane
      impression m.
    VPS (vinyl polysiloxane)
      impression m.
    wash impression m.
    ZOE-B&T base and
      temporary filling m.

Ma·thieu
    M. needle holder

mat·ri·cal

ma·tri·ces

ma·tri·cial

ma·trix *pl.* ma·tri·ces
    amalgam m.
    m. band
    bony m.
    custom m.
    dentin m.
    direct porcelain m.
    functional m.
    m. holder
    PermaRidge alveolar ridge
      hydroxylapatite m.
    platinum m.
    resin m.
    m. retainer
    silicone m.

ma·trix *(continued)*
    T-band m.

max·il·la *pl.* max·il·lae, max·
    il·las
    inferior m.

max·il·lary

max·il·lec·to·my

max·il·lo·den·tal

max·il·lo·man·dib·u·lar

max·il·lot·o·my

Max-I-Probe ir·ri·ga·tor

Max re·stor·a·tive pin

Mayne
    M. muscle control
        appliance
    M. space maintainer

Ma·yo
    M. scissors
    M.-Hegar needle holder

Ma·zot·ti
    M. reaction

MBG
    modified Boley gauge

Meck·el
    M's cave
    M.-Gruber syndrome

Med·i·cal Im·pair·ment Bu·
    reau

med·i·cine
    oral m.

med·i·co·den·tal

me·di·um *pl.* me·dia, me·
    di·ums
    disclosing m.
    separating m.

mega·karyo·cyte

Mej·char
    Edlan-M. procedure

mel·a·no·ac·an·tho·ma
    oral m.

mel·a·no·ma

mel·a·not·ic

Mel·kers·son
    M.-Rosenthal syndrome

Mel·nick
    M.-Needles syndrome

Mel·otte
    M's metal

mem·bra·na *pl.* mem·bra·nae
    m. adamantina

mem·brane
    absorbable collagen m.
    adamantine m.
    alveolodental m.
    basement m.
    collagen-
        glycosaminoglycan/
        Silastic bilayer m.
    dentinoenamel m.
    enamel m.
    Hannover's intermediate
        m.
    mucous m's
    Nasmyth's m.
    peridental m.
    periodontal m.
    poly-(L-lactic) acid m.
    polytetrafluorethylene m.
    semipermeable m.
    synovial m., inferior
    synovial m., superior

Mem·o·sil bite reg·is·tra·tion
    ma·te·ri·al

men·is·cec·to·my

me·nis·cus *pl.* me·nis·ci
    m. of temporomaxillary
        joint

Me·nis·cus Mend·er II

Me·nis·cus Mend·er nee·dle

meno·gin·gi·vi·tis
    periodic transitory m.

men·ton

me·per·i·dine

Me·piv·i·caine hy·dro·chlo·
    ride

mer·cu·ry
    dental m.

Me·ri·am cot·ton pli·ers

Mer·ri·field
    M's knife

Mer·shon
    M. arch

me·sal

mes·en·chy·mal

mesh
    polyurethane-coated
        Dacron m.
    TiMesh titanium m.
    titanium m.

me·si·al

me·si·al·ly

me·sio·buc·cal

me·sio·buc·co-oc·clu·sal

me·sio·buc·co·pul·pal

me·sio·cer·vi·cal

me·sio·cli·na·tion

me·sio·clu·sion

me·sio·dens

me·sio·dis·tal

me·sio·gin·gi·val

me·sio·in·ci·so·dis·tal

me·sio·la·bi·al

me·sio·la·bio·in·ci·sal

me·sio·lin·gual

me·sio·lin·guo·in·ci·sal

me·sio·lin·guo-oc·clu·sal

me·sio·lin·guo·pul·pal

me·si·o-oc·clu·sal

me·si·o-oc·clu·sion

me·si·o-oc·clu·so·dis·tal

me·sio·pul·pal

me·sio·pul·po·la·bi·al

me·sio·pul·po·lin·gual

me·sio·ver·sion

mes·odont

mes·odon·tic

mes·odon·tism

mes·og·nath·ic

me·sog·na·thous

meso·staph·y·line

meso·tau·ro·don·tism

Mes·ser·ann
    M. kit

Mes·sing
    M. gun

mes·uran·ic

4-META ad·he·sive res·in

meta·cone

meta·con·id

meta·con·ule

met·al
    Babbitt m.
    base m.
    basic m.
    bell m.
    cast m.
    counterdie m.
    fusible m.
    Melotte's m.
    noble m.

met·al *(continued)*
  precious m.
  white m.
  wrought m.

me·tal-ce·ram·ics

me·tal·lic

met·al·lized

met·al·liz·ing

meta·pla·sia
  chondromatous m.
  osseous m.
  m. of pulp

meta·stat·ic

meth·ac·ry·late
  polymethyl m.

meth·a·cy·cline

meth·od
  AO/ASIF m's
  Bass' m. of toothbrushing
  Callahan m.
  Charters' m. of
    toothbrushing
  chloropercha m.
  crevicular m. of
    toothbrushing
  diffusion m.
  Fones' m. of toothbrushing
  Gillies m.
  Johnson m.
  lateral condensation root
    canal filling m.
  modified Stillman's m. of
    toothbrushing
  multiple cone root canal
    filling m.
  physiologic of m. of
    toothbrushing
  retrofilling m.
  retrograde root canal
    filling m.
  root-end filling m.
  scrub-brush m. of
    toothbrushing

meth·od *(continued)*
  sectional root canal filling
    m.
  segmentation root canal
    filling m.
  silver point (cone) root
    canal filling m.
  single cone root canal
    filling m.
  split cast m.
  Stillman's m. of
    toothbrushing
  Taggard's m.
  vertical condensation root
    canal filling m.
  wash m.

meth·o·hex·i·tal

meth·o·trex·ate

meth·oxy·flu·rane

meth·yl·meth·ac·ry·late

meth·yl·pred·ni·so·lone

meth·yl·sal·i·cyl·ate

me·tro·ni·da·zole

mez·lo·cil·lin

MF-Y gold

MGC
  machinable glass ceramic

MHN
  Mohs hardness number

MI
  maximum intercuspation

Mich·i·gan "O" round probe

mi·con·a·zole

mi·cro·beads

Mi·cro·coc·cus
  M. luteus

mi·cro·don·tia

mi·cro·glos·sia

mi·cro·gna·thia

mi·cro·leak·age

Mi·cro· Plus ti·ta·ni·um plat·ing sys·tem

mi·cro·rough·ness

mi·cro·so·mia
Goldenhar hemifacial m.
hemifacial m.

mi·cro·sto·mia

Mi·cro-Vent den·tal im·plant

Mi·cro-Vent dou·ble cut·ting drill

mid·az·o·lam

mid·face

mid·line

Mier·a·dent 70

Mie·tens
M. syndrome

mi·graine

mi·gra·tion
physiologic mesial m.
tooth m., pathologic
tooth m., physiologic

Mik·u·licz
M. disease

mill
bone m.

Mil·lard
M. procedure

Mil·ler
M's elevator
M. bone file
M. curet
M. syndrome
M.-Colburn file
M.-Dieker syndrome

Mill·er Apexo el·e·va·tor

mill·ing-in

Mil·tex N-Tra·lig In·tra·lig·a·men·ta·ry An·es·the·sia Sy·ringe

Mini Five Cu·rettes

mini·plate
compression m.

mini·screws
AO m.

Mini Wrz·burg ti·ta·ni·um plat·ing sys·tem

Min·ne·so·ta re·trac·tor

mi·no·cy·cline

Min·ute Stain

Mir·a·cast al·loy

Mir·a·cle Mix core ma·te·ri·al

Mir·a·cle Mix re·stor·a·tive

Mi·rage-Bond bond·ing sys·tem

Mi·rage Plus bond·ing sys·tem

mir·ror
concave m.
convex m.
dental m.
frontal m.
head m.
mouth m.

mi·to·my·cin
m. C

mit·ra·my·cin

mix

mix·er
amalgam m.

mix·ing
vacuum m.

Mixo·mat mix·ing unit

mix·ture

MMF
   maxillomandibular fixation

MNTI
   melanotic neuroectodermal
      tumor of infancy

MO
   mesio-occlusal

mo·bil·i·ty
   abnormal tooth m.
   normal tooth m.
   pathologic tooth m.
   physiologic tooth m.
   tooth m.

mo·bil·om·e·ter

MO (mesio-occlusal) cav·i·ty

MOD
   mesio-occlusodistal

MOD (mesio-occlusodistal) cav·
   i·ty

mod·el

mod·i·fi·er
   color m.
   glass m.

Mod·u·lay al·loy

mod·u·lus
   m. of elasticity
   m. of resilience
   shear m.

Moe·bi·us
   M. sequence

Mohr
   M. syndrome

Mohs
   M. hardness number
      (MHN)
   M. hardness scale
   M. hardness test
   M. index

mo·lar
   anchor m.

mo·lar *(continued)*
   m. band
   first m.
   fourth m.
   m. hook
   impacted m.
   Moon's m's
   mulberry m.
   second m.
   sixth-year m.
   supernumerary m.
   third m.
   twelfth-year m.

mo·lar·i·form

mo·la·ris
   m. tertius

mold
   Bioblend artificial anterior
      tooth m's
   ovoid m.
   square-ovoid m.
   square-tapering-ovoid m.
   tapering-ovoid m.

mold·ing
   border m.
   compression m.
   injection m.
   tissue m.

Mol·lo·plast-B den·ture re·line

mol·lus·cum
   m. contagiosum

Molt
   M. curet
   M. elevator
   M. mouth gag
   M. periosteal elevator

mo·ment
   bending m.
   maximum bending m.

Mon·a·han
   M.-Lewis knife

mon·an·gle

Mono·gram II al·loy

Mono·gram III al·loy

mono·max·il·lary

mono·mor·phic

mono·nu·cle·o·sis
    infectious m.

mono·phy·odont

Mon·son
    anti-M. curve
    M. curve

Moon
    M's molar
    M's teeth

Moore
    M's mandrel

Moore·head
    M's retractor

Moor·hof
    Mosetig-M. filling

Mor·gan
    M's mandrel

Mor·quio
    M's syndrome

Mor·ris
    Joe Hall M. external
      skeletal pin fixation
      device

mor·sal

mor·si·ca·tio

Mo·set·ig
    M.-Moorhof filling

Moss
    M. functional matrix
      theory

mot·tling

mou·lage
    facial m.

mould

mount
    split cast m.

mount·ing
    split cast m.

mouth
    denture sore m.
    trench m.

mouth·rinse
    Peroxyl m.
    Prevention m.

mouth·stick

mouth·wash

move·ment
    Bennett m.
    bodily m. of tooth
    border m.
    border tissue m's
    buccal m.
    cutting m.
    distal m.
    envelope of border m's
    excursive m's
    free mandibular m.
    functional mandibular m.
    gliding m.
    grinding m.
    hinge m.
    intermediary m's
    intermediate m's
    jaw m.
    lingual m.
    Magnan's m.
    mandibular m.
    mandibular m., free
    mandibular m's, functional
    masticatory m's
    mesial m.
    opening m.
    opening m., posterior
    opening mandibular m.
    orthodontic tooth m.
    pendulum m's
    perverted mandibular m.
    posterior border tissue m.
    rotational m.

move·ment *(continued)*
    tipping m. of tooth
    tooth m.
    uniaxial m.

Mow·rey 695 amal·gam al·loy

Mow·rey B in·lay

Mow·rey 120 gold al·loy

Mow·rey No. 8 gold al·loy

Mow·rey S-1 gold al·loy

Mow·rey S-3 gold al·loy

Mow·rey 12% wire

Mow·rey No. 1 wire

MPS dia·mond pol·ish·ing sys·tem

MQ ce·ment

M-type ream·er

mu·ci·no·sis
    focal oral m.

mu·co·cele

mu·co·ep·i·der·moid

mu·co·gin·gi·val

mu·co·poly·sac·cha·ri·do·sis

mu·cor·my·co·sis

mu·co·sa
    buccal m.
    palatal m.

mu·co·stat·ic

mud
    dentin m.

muf·fle

Mühle·mann
    M. appliance

mull·ing

mul·ti·cus·pid

mul·ti·cus·pi·date

Mul·ti·form du·al pur·pose im·pres·sion paste

mul·ti·root·ed
al pur·pose

mumps

MURCS as·so·ci·a·tion

mus·cle
    Aeby's m.
    Albinus' m.
    anterior digastric m.
    buccinator m.
    buccopharyngeal m.
    canine m.
    cheek m.
    chondroglossus m.
    constrictor m's of pharynx
    constrictor m. of pharynx, inferior
    constrictor m. of pharynx, middle
    constrictor m. of pharynx, superior
    depressor m. of angle of mouth
    depressor m. of lower lip
    digastric m.
    facial m's
    m's of facial expression
    facial and masticatory m's
    m's of fauces
    genioglossus m.
    geniohyoid m.
    glossopalatine m.
    glossopharyngeal m.
    hyoglossal m.
    hyoglossus m.
    incisive m's of inferior lip
    incisive m's of lower lip
    incisive m's of superior lip
    incisive m's of upper lip
    infrahyoid m's
    levator m. of angle of mouth
    levator anguli oris m.
    levator labii superioris alaeque nasi m.

mus·cle *(continued)*
    levator labii superioris m.
    levator m. of upper lip
    levator m. of upper lip and
      ala of nose
    levator veli palatini m.
    lingual m's
    masseter m.
    m's of mastication
    masticatory m's
    mentalis m.
    mylohyoid m.
    mylopharyngeal m.
    orbicular m. of mouth
    orbicularis oris m.
    m's of palate and fauces
    palatine m's
    palatoglossus m.
    palatopharyngeal m.
    pharyngopalatine m.
    platysma m.
    pterygoid m., external
    pterygoid m., internal
    pterygoid m., lateral
    pterygoid m., medial
    pterygopharyngeal m.
    quadrate m. of lower lip
    quadrate m. of upper lip
    risorius m.
    salpingopharyngeal m.
    Santorini's m.
    styloglossus m.
    stylohyoid m.
    stylopharyngeus m.
    suprahyoid m's
    temporal m.
    temporalis m's
    tensor m. of velum palatini
    tensor veli palatini m.
    m's of tongue
    transverse m. of chin
    transverse m. of tongue
    zygomatic m.
    zygomatic m., greater
    zygomatic m., lesser

mus·cu·lus *pl.* mus·cu·li
    m. buccinator

mus·cu·lus *(continued)*
    m. buccopharyngeus
    m. caninus
    m. chondroglossus
    m. constrictor pharyngis
      inferior
    m. constrictor pharyngis
      medius
    m. constrictor pharyngis
      superior
    m. depressor anguli oris
    m. depressor labii
      inferioris
    m. digastricus
    musculi faciales et
      masticatores
    m. genioglossus
    m. geniohyoideus
    m. glossopalatinus
    m. glossopharyngeus
    m. hyoglossus
    musculi incisivi labii
      inferioris
    musculi incisivi labii
      superioris
    m. levator anguli oris
    m. levator labii superioris
    m. levator labii superioris
      alaeque nasi
    musculi linguae
    m. masseter
    m. mylohyoideus
    m. mylopharyngeus
    m. orbicularis oris
    musculi palati
    musculi palati et faucium
    m. palatoglossus
    m. palatopharyngeus
    m. pharyngopalatinus
    m. pterygoideus externus
    m. pterygoideus internus
    m. pterygoideus lateralis
    m. pterygoideus medialis
    m. pterygopharyngeus
    m. quadratus labii
      inferioris
    m. quadratus labii
      superioris

mus·cu·lus *(continued)*
   m. risorius
   m. salpingopharyngeus
   m. styloglossus
   m. stylohyoideus
   m. stylopharyngeus
   musculi suprahyoidei
   m. temporalis
   m. tensor veli palatini
   m. transversus linguae
   m. transversus menti
   m. zygomaticus
   m. zygomaticus major
   m. zygomaticus minor

my·al·gia

my·as·the·nia
   m. gravis

my·co·sis
   m. fungoides

my·elo·ma
   multiple m.

my·e·lo·per·ox·i·dase (MPO)

My·nol ce·ment

myo·func·tion·al

Myo-Mon·i·tor cen·tric

myo·si·tis
   proliferative m.

myo·spher·u·lo·sis

Myrrh & Ben·zoin Tinc·ture

myx·o·ma *pl.* myx·o·mas, myx·o·ma·ta
   odontogenic m.

myxo·sar·co·ma
   m. of nerve sheath

Na·bers
    N. probe

Na·ger
    N. syndrome

Nance
    N. holding arch
    N's leeway space

na·si·on

Nas·myth
    N's membrane

na·so·al·ve·o·lar

na·so·pal·a·tine

na·so·pha·ryn·ge·al

na·tal

na·vel
    enamel n.

Nd:YAG
    neodymium:yttrium-
      aluminum-garnet

Nd:YAG (neodymium:yttrium-
    aluminum-garnet) la·ser

Nea·lon
    N's technique

Nebs an·al·ge·sic li·quid

neck
    n. of condyloid process of
      mandible
    dental n.
    n. of mandible
    n. of tooth

ne·crol·y·sis
    toxic epidermal n.

ne·cro·sis *pl.* ne·cro·ses
    alar n.
    bone n.
    caseation n.

ne·cro·sis *(continued)*
    caseous n.
    cheesy n.
    coagulation n.
    coagulative n.
    colliquative n.
    dry n.
    epiphyseal ischemic n.
    exanthematous n.
    focal n.
    gangrenous n.
    gangrenous pulp n.
    injection n.
    ischemic n.
    liquefaction n.
    liquefactive n.
    moist n.
    phosphorus n.

ne·crot·ic

nec·ro·tiz·ing

nee·dle
    Atraloc n.
    compound curved tapercut
      n.
    endodontic n.
    French spring eye n.
    Lane cleft palate n.
    Meniscus Mender n.
    point cut n.
    reverse cutting n.

Nee·dles
    Melnick-N. syndrome

Nee·dle Tubes

Nem·bu·tal

Neo·co·bef·rin

neo·dy·mi·um:YAG (yttrium-
    aluminum-garnet) la·ser

neo·na·tal

neo·pla·sia
    multiple endocrine n. type III

neo·plasm
    malignant neurogenous n.

Neo-Plex im·pres·sion ma·te·ri·al

neo·spor·in

Neo-Temp ce·ment

Neo·Wax base·plate wax

nerve
    abducens n.
    alveolar n.
    alveolar n., inferior
    alveolar n's, superior
    anterior palatine n.
    anterior superior alveolar n.
    auriculotemporal n.
    Bock's n.
    buccal n.
    buccinator n.
    cranial n's
    dental n., inferior
    ethmoid n.
    glossopharyngeal n.
    greater palatine n.
    hypoglossal n.
    inferior alveolar n.
    inferior dental n.
    laryngeal n.
    lingual n.
    mandibular n.
    masseteric n.
    masticator n.
    maxillary n.
    mental n.
    middle meningeal n.
    middle superior alveolar n.
    mylohyoid n.
    ophthalmic n.
    palatine n., anterior
    palatine n., greater
    palatine n's, lesser
    palatine n's, medial

nerve *(continued)*
    palatine n's, middle
    palatine n., posterior
    posterior superior alveolar n.
    trigeminal n.

ner·vus *pl.* ner·vi
    n. alveolaris inferior
    nervi alveolares superiores
    n. buccalis
    n. buccinatorius
    nervi craniales
    n. glossopharyngeus
    n. hypoglossus
    n. lingualis
    n. mandibularis
    n. massetericus
    n. masticatorius
    n. maxillaris
    n. mentalis
    n. mylohyoideus
    nervi palatini
    n. palatinus anterior
    n. palatinus major
    n. palatinus medius
    nervi palatini minores
    n. palatinus posterior
    nervi terminales
    n. trigeminus

Neu
    N.-Laxova syndrome

Neu·mann
    N. sheath
    sheath of N.

neu·ral

neu·ral·gia
    glossopharyngeal n.
    mandibular joint n.
    Sluder's n.
    sphenopalatine n.
    trigeminal n.

neu·ri·le·mo·ma
    malignant n.

neu·ri·no·ma
  malignant n.

neu·ro·blas·to·ma

neu·ro·ec·to·der·mal

neu·ro·fi·bro·ma

neu·ro·fi·bro·ma·to·sis

neu·ro·fi·bro·sar·co·ma

Neu·rohr
  N. spring-lock attachment
  N.-Williams rest shoe

neu·ro·lem·mo·ma

neu·ro·ma
  amputation n.
  traumatic n.

neu·rop·a·thy
  isolated, nontraumatic
    mental branch n. (IMNN)

neu·ro·the·ke·o·ma
  intraoral n.

neu·tro·clu·sion

neu·tro·pe·nia
  cyclic n.

Ne·vi·us
  N. forceps

ne·vo·cel·lu·lar

ne·void

ne·vus *pl.* ne·vi
  blue n.
  compound n.
  intramucosal n.
  junctional n.
  nevocellular n.
  Spitz n.
  white sponge n.

Ney ar·tic·u·la·tor

Ney-Oro al·loy

Ney sur·vey·or

nib

niche
  enamel n.

nick·el

nic·o·tine

ni·gri·cans

nip·pers
  Goldman-Fox n.
  Sugarman Nipro n.

ni·trous
  n. oxide

No·bel·phar·ma en·dos·se·ous
  im·plants

No·bil·li·um al·loy

node
  buccal lymph n.
  lymph n.
  mandibular lymph n.
  maxillary lymph n's
  subdigastric n's
  submandibular lymph n's
  submental lymph n's
  subparotid lymph n's
  suprahyoid lymph n's
  tonsillar lymph n's

nod·ule
  Bohn's n's
  enamel n.
  pulp n.
  secondary n.

NO·gen·ol bite reg·is·tra·tion
  paste

NO·gen·ol ce·ment

NO·gen·ol root ca·nal seal·er

no·ma

non-Hodg·kin's lym·pho·ma

non·oc·clu·sion

Noo·nan
  N's syndrome

Nord
    N. appliance
    N. expansion plate
    N. plate

no·ta·tion
    Palmer n.

notch
    hamular n.
    labial n.
    lacrimal n. of maxilla
    mandibular n.
    semilunar n. of mandible
    sigmoid n. of mandible

NSAIA
    nonsteroidal anti-
        inflammatory agent

NSAID
    nonsteroidal anti-
        inflammatory drug

nu·cle·us *pl.* nu·clei
    dental n.

Nu Gauze sponge

Nu-Lite re·trac·tor

num·ber
    Brinell hardness n.
    hardness n.
    Knoop hardness n.

num·ber *(continued)*
    Mohs hardness n.
    Rockwell hardness n.
    Vickers hardness n.

NUP
    necrotizing ulcerative
        periodontitis

Nu·pro APF gel

Nu·pro flu·o·ride gel

Nu·pro Neu·tral flu·o·ride so·
    lu·tion

Nu·pro Plus pro·phy·lax·is
    paste

Nupro pro·phy·lax·is paste

Nürn·berg gold

Nu·va-Lite seal·ant

Nu·va-PA com·pos·ite res·in

Nu·va-Seal seal·ant

Nu·va-Sys·tem tooth con·di·
    tion·er

Ny·gaard
    N.-Otsby frame

nys·ta·tin

ob·tu·ra·tion
  canal o.

ob·tu·ra·tor
  Case's velum o.
  Densfil thermal endodontic
    o's

Ob·weg·es·er
  O. awl
  O. ramus retractor
  O.-Dal Pont sagittal split
    osteotomy

oc·clude

oc·clud·er

oc·clu·sal

oc·clu·sion
  abnormal o.
  acentric o.
  adjusted o.
  o. analysis
  anatomic o.
  anterior o.
  attritional o.
  balanced o.
  buccal o.
  centric o.
  centric relation o.
  convenience o.
  coronary o.
  crossbite o.
  cuspid protected o.
  distal o.
  dynamic o.
  eccentric o.
  edge-to-edge o.
  end-to-end o.
  functional o.
  gliding o.
  habitual o.
  handheld centric o.
  hyperfunctional o.
  ideal o.

oc·clu·sion *(continued)*
  labial o.
  lateral o.
  lingual o.
  locked o.
  malfunctional o.
  mechanically balanced o.
  mesial o.
  milled-in o.
  neutral o.
  normal o.
  pathogenic o.
  physiologic o.
  physiologically balanced o.
  posterior o.
  postnormal o.
  prenormal o.
  primary traumatic o.
  protrusive o.
  retrusive o.
  secondary traumatic o.
  spherical form of o.
  terminal o.
  traumatic o.
  traumatogenic o.
  working o.

oc·clu·sive

oc·clu·so·cer·vi·cal

oc·clu·som·e·ter

oc·clu·so·re·ha·bil·i·ta·tion

Och·sen·bein
  Luebke-O. flap
  O. chisel

Oc·to·caine

odon·tal·gia
  phantom o.

odon·tal·gic

odon·tec·to·my
  partial o.

odont·iat·ro·genic

odon·tic

odon·to·am·e·lo·blas·to·ma

odon·to·blast

odon·to·both·ri·on

odon·to·both·ri·tis

odon·to·cla·mis

odon·to·clast

odon·to·dys·pla·sia
    regional o.

odon·to·gen

odon·to·gen·e·sis

odon·to·ge·net·ic

odon·to·gen·ic

odon·tog·e·nous

odon·to·gram

odon·to·graph

odon·tog·ra·phy

odon·to·iat·ria

odon·tol·o·gist

odon·tol·o·gy
    forensic o.

odon·to·ma
    o. adamantinum
    ameloblastic o.
    calcified o.
    complex o.
    composite o.
    composite o., complex
    composite o., compound
    compound o.
    coronal o.
    coronary o.
    cystic o.
    cystic complex o.
    dilated o.
    embryoplastic o.
    epithelial o.

odon·to·ma *(continued)*
    fibrous o.
    gestant o.
    malignant o.
    mixed o.
    radicular o.
    soft mixed o.

odon·ton·o·my

odon·to·peri·os·te·um

odon·to·plas·ty

odon·to·pri·sis

odon·tos·co·py

odon·to·sis

odon·to·the·ca

odon·tot·o·my

OHI-S
    Simplified Oral Hygiene
    Index

Ohl
    O. elevator

oil
    o. of cloves

oligo·don·tia

Oli·ver
    Adams-O. syndrome
    O. pliers

Ol·sen
    O. stiffness tester
    O.-Hegar needle holder

Olym·pia al·loy

Om·ni·flex im·pres·sion ma·
    te·ri·al

Om·ni·loc im·plant

OMS
    Oral and Maxillofacial
    Surgeons

OMSF
    Oral and Maxillofacial
    Surgery Foundation

ON
    onlay

on·co·cy·to·ma

on·co·cy·to·sis

On·yx L/G Black Etch

Op
    opisthocranion

opa·ci·fi·er

opal·es·cence

opal·es·cent

opaqu·er
    Goldlink O.

O-PDS
    O-Polydioxanone suture

open·er
    bite o.
    dynamic bite o.
    orifice o.

open·ing
    interincisal o.

op·er·a·tion
    Billroth's o.
    Brophy's o.
    Caldwell-Luc o.
    Commando's o.
    Fergusson's o.
    flap o.
    Gillies o.
    Heath's o.
    Kazanjian's o.
    Kocher's o.
    Krimer's o.
    Liston's o.
    Lizars' o.
    Luc's o.
    Partsch's o.
    Regnoli's o.

op·er·a·tory

oper·cu·lec·to·my

oper·cu·li·tis

oper·cu·lum *pl.* oper·cu·la
    cartilaginous o.
    dental o.

opis·thog·na·thism

Opitz
    O. syndrome
    Smith-Lemli-O. syndrome

O-Poly·di·ox·an·one su·ture
    (O-PDS)

Op·o·tow im·pres·sion paste

Op·o·tow jaw re·la·tion rec·
    ords

Op·o·tow Jel·set im·pres·sion
    ma·te·ri·al

Op·site semi·per·me·able poly·
    ure·thane dress·ing

Op·ta·loy al·loy

Op·ti·lux 400

Op·tion al·loy

Ora·base oral pro·tec·tive
    paste

oral

Oral and Max·il·lo·fa·cial Sur·
    gery Foun·da·tion

oral·o·gy

Ora5 oral an·ti·bac·te·ri·al
    agent

Ora·stat

Or·ban
    O. file
    O. hoe scaler
    O. knife

or·bi·ta·le

or·gan
    cement o.

or·gan *(continued)*
    enamel o.
    o's of mastication

or·i·fice
    o. of pulp canal

oro·an·tral

oro·lin·gual

or·tho·den·tin

or·tho·don·tia

or·tho·don·tic

or·tho·don·tics
    camouflage o.
    corrective o.
    interceptive o.
    preventive o.
    prophylactic o.
    surgical o.

or·tho·don·tist

or·tho·don·tol·o·gy

or·thog·nath·ia

or·thog·na·thic

or·thog·na·thous

or·tho·ker·a·tin

or·tho·ker·a·tin·iza·tion

or·tho·ker·a·tin·ized

or·tho·pe·dics
    dentofacial o.
    functional jaw o.

or·tho·sis *pl.* or·tho·ses
    Vancouver microstomia o.

or·thot·ic

Or·ti·co·chea
    O. pharyngoplasty

Or·ton
    O's enamel cleaver

Or·yl den·ture lin·ing ma·te·
    ri·al

OSAS
    obstructive sleep apnea
    syndrome

OSCC
    oral squamous cell
    carcinomas

Os·seo·dent im·plant

Os·seo·dont Den·tal Im·plant
    Sys·tem

os·seo·in·te·grat·ed

os·seo·in·te·gra·tion

os·se·ous

os·si·fy·ing

os·tec·to·my
    mandibular body o.
    oblique o.
    peripheral o.

os·te·itis
    alveolar o.

os·teo·ar·thri·tis

os·teo·blast

os·teo·blas·to·ma

os·teo·ce·men·tum

os·teo·chon·dro·ma

os·teo·dys·tro·phy
    Albright's hereditary o.

os·teo·gen·e·sis
    o. imperfecta (OI)
    o. imperfecta, type I

Os·teo·Gen im·plant

Os·teo·Gen low tem·per·a·ture
    hy·droxy·ap·a·tite

Os·teo·graf/AR

Os·teo·graf/N

Os·teo·graf/P

os·te·oid

os·teo·in·duc·tion

Os·teo-Loc en·do·don·tic sta·
  bi·li·za·tion

Os·teo-Loc Plate Form Sys·tem

Os·teo-Loc Root Form Sys·tem

os·te·o·ma
  giant osteoid o.
  osteoid o.

os·teo·my·eli·tis
  acute o.
  chronic o.
  condylar o.
  dry socket o.
  Garré's o.
  sclerosing o.

os·teo·myo·cu·ta·ne·ous

os·teo·pe·nia
  stress-protected, stress-
    shielded o.

os·teo·peri·os·ti·tis
  alveolodental o.

os·teo·pe·tro·sis
  autosomal recessive–lethal
    o.

os·teo·pro·mo·tion

os·teo·ra·dio·ne·cro·sis

os·teo·sar·co·ma
  chondroblastic o.
  fibroblastic o.
  juxtacortical o.
  osteoblastic o.
  parosteal o.
  periosteal o.
  radiation-induced o.

os·teo·syn·the·sis
  bone plate o.
  bone screw–wire o.
  compression o.
  plate and screw o.
  wire o.

os·teo·tome
  spatula o.

os·te·ot·o·my
  bilateral sagittal ramus o's
  bilateral sagittal split o.
    (BSSO)
  block o.
  C o.
  C-form o.
  closed o.
  Dal Pont sagittal split o.
  extraoral vertical ramus o.
    (EVRO)
  horizontal o.
  horizontal mandibular o.
  Hunsuck sagittal split o.
  interpositional o's
  intraoral vertical ramus o.
  intraoral vertical ramus o.
    (IVRO)
  inverted-L o.
  inverted-L-form o.
  Le Fort o.
  Le Fort I o.
  Le Fort I maxillary o.
  linear o.
  mandibular o.
  maxillary step o.
  midface o.
  midpalatal o.
  Obwegeser-Dal Pont
    sagittal split o.
  parasagittal o.
  open o.
  perforation o.
  ramus o.
  sagittal ramus o.
  sagittal split o.
  sagittal split ramus o.
    (SSRO)
  sandwich o.
  sliding horizontal o.
  subapical o.
  subapical mandibular o.
  subcondylar mandibular o.
  subcondylar oblique o.
  total maxillary o.
  transoral vertical oblique
    o.
  vertical o.

os·te·ot·o·my *(continued)*
    vertical oblique ramus o.
    vertical ramus o.
    vertical o. of ramus of
      mandible
    vertical subcondylar o.
    visor o.
    visor/sandwich o.

otal·gia
    maxillary o.

Ots·by
    Nygaard-O. frame
    O. frame

O-type ream·er

oulec·to·my

ouli·tis

over·bite
    deep o.
    horizontal o.
    vertical o.

over·case

over·clo·sure
    reduced interarch distance
      o.

over·den·ture
    Flexi-Post o.
    implant-supported o.

over·erup·tion

over·growth
    gingival o.

over·hang

over·jet

over·jut

over·lap
    deep vertical o.
    horizontal o.
    vertical o.

over·lay

over·struc·ture

Owen
    line of O.

ox·a·cil·lin

Ox·a·ze·pam

ox·ide
    stannic o.

oxy·co·done

ox·yt·a·lan

ox·yt·a·lan·ol·y·sis

oxy·tet·ra·cy·cline

ozo·ce·rite

pa·chyg·na·thous

pachy·onych·ia
    p. congenita

pack
    acrylate p.
    antral p.
    eugenol p.
    Kirkland periodontal p.
    Kirkland-Kaiser p.
    periodontal p.
    periodontal noneugenol p.
    pharyngeal p.
    pressure p.
    throat p.

pad
    buccal fat p.
    fat p.
    gum p's
    lip p.
    nasolabial fat p.
    occlusal p.
    retromolar p.
    submental fat p.
    sucking p.
    suctorial p.

Pa·get
    P. disease

pain
    atypical facial p.

pal·a·tal

pal·ate
    artificial p.
    bony p.
    bony hard p.
    Byzantine p.
    cleft p.
    gothic p.
    grooved p.
    hard p.
    osseous p.
    pendulous p.

pal·ate *(continued)*
    primary p.
    secondary p.
    smoker's p.
    soft p.
    submucous cleft p.
    unilateral cleft p.

pal·a·tine

pal·a·to·plas·ty
    von Langenbeck p.
    V-Y p.

pal·a·to·prox·i·mal

Pal·gin·ex 75 im·pres·sion ma·te·ri·al

pal·la·di·um

Pal·lis·ter
    P.-Hall syndrome

Pal·mer
    P. notation

pal·sy
    Bell's p.
    facial p.

Pa·na·via Den·tal Ad·he·sive

Pa·na·via lut·ing ce·ment

pan·cu·ro·ni·um bro·mide

pan·to·graph

pa·per
    Articodent articulating p.
    articulating p.

pa·pil·la *pl.* pa·pil·lae
    interdental p.
    interproximal p.
    palatine p.
    retromolar p.
    sublingual p.

pap·il·lary

pa·pil·lif·er·um

pap·il·lo·ma

Pa·pil·lon
   P.-Lefevre syndrome

para·cone

para·co·nid

para·den·tal

para·den·ti·tis

para·den·ti·um

para·den·to·sis

par·af·fin

para·gan·gli·o·ma

Par·a·gon acryl·ic res·in

para·ker·a·tin

par·al·lel·om·e·ter

Par·a·max II par·al·lel·om·e·
  ter

Para Post sys·tem

para·rhi·zo·cla·sia

para·sym·phy·sis
   mandibular p.

para·zone

par·es·the·sia

pa·rot·i·de·an

pa·rot·i·dec·to·my

par·oti·tis
   chronic obstructive p.
    (COP)
   recurrent p.
   recurrent p. in childhood
    (RPC)

pars *pl.* par·tes
   p. alaris musculi nasalis
   p. alveolaris mandibulae
   p. amorpha
   p. basilaris ossis occipitalis

pars *(continued)*
   p. buccopharyngea musculi
    constrictoris pharyngis
    superioris
   p. cartilaginea septi nasi
   p. ceratopharyngea
    musculi constrictoris
    pharyngis medii
   p. cervicalis systematis
    sympathici
   p. chondropharyngea
    musculi constrictoris
    pharyngis medii
   p. cochlearis nervi octavi,
    p.
   p. cochlearis nervi
    vestibulocochlearis
   partes corporis humani
   p. cricopharyngea musculi
    constrictoris pharyngis
    inferioris
   p. glossopharyngea
    musculi constrictoris
    pharyngis superioris
   p. horizontalis ossis
    palatini
   p. infundibularis lobi
    anterioris hypophyseos
   p. intercartilaginea rimae
    glottidis
   p. intermembranacea
    rimae glottidis
   p. labialis musculi
    orbicularis oris
   p. lacrimalis musculi
    orbicularis oculi
   p. laryngea pharyngis
   p. lateralis ossis occipitalis
   p. marginalis musculi
    orbicularis oris
   p. mastoidea ossis
    temporalis
   p. membranacea septi nasi
   p. mobilis septi nasi
   p. mylopharyngea musculi
    constrictoris pharyngis
    superioris
   p. nasalis ossis frontalis

pars *(continued)*
    p. nasalis pharyngis
    p. nervosa hypophyseos
    p. obliqua musculi
        cricothyroidei
    p. oralis pharyngis
    p. orbitalis musculi
        orbicularis oculi
    p. orbitalis ossis frontalis
    p. ossea septi nasi
    p. palpebralis glandulae
        lacrimalis
    p. palpebralis musculi
        orbicularis oculi
    p. parasympathica
        systematis nervosi
        autonomici
    p. perpendicularis ossis
        palatini
    p. petrosa ossis temporalis
    p. profunda glandulae
        parotideae
    p. profunda musculi
        masseteris
    p. pterygopharyngea
        musculi constrictoris
        pharyngis superioris
    p. squamosa ossis
        temporalis
    p. superficialis musculi
        masseteris
    p. sympathetica systematis
        nervosi autonomici
    p. thyropharyngea musculi
        constrictoris pharyngis
        inferioris
    p. transversa musculi
        nasalis
    p. tympanica ossis
        temporalis

part
    alar p. of nasalis muscle
    alveolar p. of mandible
    basilar p. of occipital bone
    bony p. of nasal septum
    condylar p. of occipital
        bone

part *(continued)*
    cranial p. of accessory
        nerve
    deep p. of parotid gland
    exoccipital p. of occipital
        bone
    jugular p. of occipital bone
    lateral p. of occipital bone
    mamillary p. of temporal
        bone
    membranous p. of nasal
        septum
    occipital p. of occipital
        bone
    palpebral p. of lacrimal
        gland
    squamous p. of occipital
        bone
    squamous p. of temporal
        bone

Partsch
    P's operation

pa·ru·lis

PAS
    periodic acid–Schiff

Pas·cord re·trac·tion cord

Pas·sa·vant
    P's bar

pas·ser
    foil p.

pas·siv·i·ty

paste
    Abbot's p.
    base p.
    benzocaine dental p.
    Blu-Mousse impression p.
    bone p.
    Caulk impression p.
    Cinch-Vinyl vinyl
        polysiloxane impression
        material p.
    Coe-Flo impression p.
    Coe-Pak p.
    denture p.

paste *(continued)*

    denture adherent p.
    desensitizing p.
    fibrin-collagen p.
    filler p.
    Glossy polishing p.
    Gum-Aid analgesic p.
    Hydent denture indicator
      p.
    Hypo-Cal calcium
      hydroxide p.
    Insta-Glaze polishing p.
    Kerr equalizing p.
    Lassar's p.
    Luralite impression p.
    luster p.
    Magnasil prophylaxis p.
    metallic oxide p.
    Multiform dual purpose
      impression p.
    Multiform impression p.
    NOgenol bite registration
      p.
    noneugenol p.
    Nupro Plus prophylaxis p.
    Nupro prophylaxis p.
    Opotow impression p.
    Orabase oral protective p.
    Plastopaste impression p.
    polishing p.
    pressure indicator p.
    Pro-Care prophylaxis p.
    pumice p.
    Sergenti p.
    sodium flouride p.
    Super Bite bite
      registration p.
    Superpaste impression p.
    Temp-Canal p.
    tooth p.
    Topex prophylaxis p.
    Uni-Pro prophylaxis p.
    Wachs p.
    zinc oxide p.
    zinc oxide and eugenol p.
    zinc oxide–eugenol
      impression p.
    Zircate prophylaxis p.

paste *(continued)*

    Zircon F prophylaxis p.
    Ziroxide prophylaxis p.
    ZOE (zinc oxide–eugenol)
      impression p.

path

    centric p. of closure
    condyle p.
    generated occlusal p.
    idling p.
    incisor p.
    p. of insertion
    lateral condyle p.
    milled-in p's
    occlusal p.
    occlusal p., generated
    p. of placement
    protrusive condyle p.
    p. of removal
    working p.

path·find·er

Path·find·er CS

path·odon·tia

pa·thol·o·gist
    oral p.

pa·thol·o·gy
    dental p.
    oral p.

path·way
    lipoxygenase p.

pa·tient
    immunocompromised p's

pat·tern
    investing the p.
    occlusal p.
    trabecular p.
    wax p.
    wear p.

Pat·tern acryl·ic res·in

Paul·us ti·ta·ni·um chin plate
    sys·tem

Paul·us ti·ta·ni·um plat·ing sys·tem

P-10 com·pos·ite res·in

P-30 com·pos·ite res·in

Péan
  Rochester-P. hemostat

pearl
  enamel p's
  Epstein's p's

Peck
  P's purple hard wax

pe·dio·don·tia

pe·do·don·tia

pe·do·don·tics

pe·do·don·tist

Pee·so
  P. drill
  P. pliers
  P. reamers

pel·let
  foil p.
  cotton p's
  Epidri p's
  gold foil p.

pel·li·cle
  enamel p.
  dental p's

pem·phi·goid
  bullous p.
  mucous membrane p.

pem·phi·gus

Pe·na
  P.-Shokeir phenotype

pen·i·cil·lin
  p. G
  p. G procaine
  phenoxymethyl p.
  p. V

Pen·rose
  P. drain

pen·to·bar·bi·tal

Pen·to·thal

pen·to·thal so·di·um

Pep·to·coc·cus

Pep·to·strep·to·coc·cus
  P. anaerobius

Per·fex re·pair res·in

per·fo·ra·tion
  impression p.
  tooth p.

Per·fourm Hy·dro·ac·tiv im·pres·sion ma·te·ri·al

peri·apex

peri·ap·i·cal

peri·ce·men·tal

peri·ce·men·ti·tis
  apical p.
  chronic suppurative p.

peri·ce·men·tum

peri·cor·o·nal

peri·cor·o·ni·tis

peri·den·tal

peri·den·ti·um

Per·i·dex

peri-im·plan·to·cla·sia
  exfoliative p.
  necrotic ulcerative p.
  resorption p.
  traumatic p.
  ulcerative p.

peri·ky·ma·ta *sing.* peri·ky·ma

pe·rim·e·ter
  dental p.

Peri·o·care peri·odon·tal
  dress·ing

peri·odon·tal

peri·odon·tia

peri·odon·tics

peri·odon·tist

peri·odon·ti·tis
    adult p.
    apical p.
    chronic apical p.
    juvenile p.
    marginal p.
    necrotizing ulcerative p.
      (NUP)
    prepubertal p.
    rapidly progressive p.
    simple p.
    p. simplex

peri·odon·to·cla·sia

peri·odon·tol·o·gy

peri·odon·to·sis

peri·oral

Peri·o·SE·LECT flu·o·ride gel

Perio·SE·LECT perio·rinse

peri·os·teo·tome

peri·os·te·um
    alveolar p.
    p. alveolare

Perio·test

per·ox·i·dase
    salivary p.

Peri·pac peri·odon·tal pack·
  ing ma·te·ri·al

pe·riph·er·al

peri·ra·dic·u·lar

peri·rhi·zo·cla·sia

Per·ma·Bond al·loy

Per·ma·dyne Gar·ant im·pres·
  sion ma·te·ri·al

Per·ma·dyne im·pres·sion ma·
  te·ri·al

Per·ma·gum Gar·ant im·pres·
  sion ma·te·ri·al

Per·ma·gum im·pres·sion ma·
  te·ri·al

Per·ma·Ridge al·ve·o·lar ridge
  hy·drox·yl·ap·a·tite ma·trix

Perm·las·tic im·pres·sion ma·
  te·ri·al

per·ni·cious

Per·ox·ide

Per·ox·yl gel

Per·ry
    Darby-P. scaler
    P. cotton pliers

Per·tac Uni·ver·sal Bond bond·
  ing sys·tem

Peutz
    P.-Jeghers syndrome

Pfeif·fer
    P's syndrome

PFM
    porcelain-fused-to-metal

PFM crown

PGA
    polyglycolic acid

phar·yn·gi·tis
    lymphonodular p.

pha·ryn·go·plas·ty
    Orticochea p.

Phen·er·gan

phe·no·bar·bi·tal

phe·no·type
    Pena-Shokeir p.

phen·oxy·meth·yl pen·i·cil·lin

phen·yl·eph·rine

phen·y·to·in

pho·na·tion

Pho·to·bond bond·ing sys·tem

phys·i·ol·o·gy
dental p.

PI
periodontal index
plaque index

pick
apical p.
crane p.
Heidbrink root p.
Heidbrink root-tip p.
Howard apexo root p.
Potts root p.
root p.

Pick·er·ill
P's imbrication line

pick·ler

pick·ling

pier

Pi·erre Ro·bin
P.R. anomalad
P.R. syndrome

pig·men·ta·tion
amalgam tattoo p.
chloroquine p.
exogenous p.

pi·mo·zide

pin
Bondent dentin bonding p.
cemented p.
channel shoulder p. (CSP)
endodontic p.
friction p.
friction-retained p.
incisal p.
incisal guide p.
Kirschner p's
Max restorative p.

pin *(continued)*
retention p.
Roger-Anderson p.
screw p.
self-threading p.
Stabilok dental p.
Steinmann p.
Thread Timed Transfer P's
TMS (thread mate system)
p.
TMS Link Plus retention
p.

Pin-Dal·bo at·tach·ment

Pind·borg
P. tumor

pin·ledge

pip·er·a·cil·lin

pit
commissural lip p's
paramedian lip p's
pterygoid p.

pi·tu·i·tary

piv·ot
adjustable occlusal p.
occlusal p.

P.K. Tho·mas
P.K.T. waxing instrument

place·ment
lingual p.

Plac·i·dyl

pla·gio·ceph·a·ly
anterior p.

plane
axiolabiolingual p.
axiomesiodistal p.
base p.
bite p.
buccolingual p.
cusp p.
guide p.
guiding p.
horizontal p.

plane *(continued)*
 labiolingual p.
 mean foundation p.
 mesiodistal p.
 occlusal p.
 p. of occlusion
 tooth p.
 transverse p. of space

plan·ing
 root p.

plaque
 bacterial p.
 dental p.

plas·ma·cy·to·ma
 solitary p. of bone

plas·ter
 dental p.
 Hapset hydroxyapatite
  bone graft p.
 impression p.
 lab p.
 model p.
 p. of Paris

plas·tic
 modeling p.
 molding p.
 synthetic p.

plas·tic·i·ty

plas·ti·ci·zer

Plas·to·dent elas·tic im·pres·sion pow·der

Plas·to·paste im·pres·sion paste

plas·to·quin·one

plate
 AO p.
 AO mandibular
  reconstruction p.
 AO/ASIF reconstruction p.
 bandelette p.
 base p.
 basic p.
 bite p.

plate *(continued)*
 bone p.
 Champy p's
 Coffin p.
 Coffin split p.
 compression p.
 cortical p.
 cribriform p. of alveolar
  process
 dental p.
 die p.
 dynamic compression p.
 expansion p.
 Hawley bite p.
 horizontal p. of palatine
  bone
 Howmedica dynamic
  compression p.
 jumping the bite p.
 Kingsley p.
 Lane p's
 lingual p.
 low-profile titanium p.
 mandibular staple bone p.
 metal p's
 micro titanium p.
 mini dynamic compression
  p.
 mini titanium p.
 noncompression
  monocortical p's
 Nord p.
 Nord expansion p.
 orthotic bite p.
 palatal p.
 palate p.
 Paulus chin p.
 reconstruction p.
 Sherman p.
 six-hole reconstruction p.
 split p.
 spring p.
 Steinhäuser p's
 Synthes dynamic
  compression p.
 three-dimensional,
  bendable reconstruction
  p. (3-DBRP)

plate *(continued)*
    3-D titanium p.
    titanium p's
    Würzburg titanium
      condylar p.
    Y p.

plat·ing
    bone p.
    gold p.

Pla·ti·nore al·loy

platy·staph·y·line

Plaut
    P.-Vincent infection

Plax den·tal rinse

Plea·sure
    P. curve

pleo·mor·phic

plex·i·form

plex·us *pl.* plex·us, plex·us·es
    p. of Raschkow

pli·ers
    Abell p.
    Aderer p.
    Allen's root p.
    back-action cotton p.
    band p.
    band-removing p.
    bird beak bending p.
    clasp bending p.
    college cotton p.
    contouring p.
    corn suture p.
    cotton p.
    cusp forming p.
    cutting p.
    eagle's beak p.
    elastic inserting p.
    endodontic p.
    Fischer p.
    flat nose p.
    foil p.
    foil carrying p.
    Gordon p.

pli·ers *(continued)*
    How p.
    How crown p.
    Jarabak p.
    Johnson p.
    ligature cutting p.
    ligature tying p.
    locking cotton p.
    McKellop p.
    matrix p.
    Meriam cotton p.
    non-pinch cotton p.
    Oliver p.
    orthodontic p.
    Peeso p.
    Perry cotton p.
    Reynolds p.
    round p.
    self-locking cotton p.
    serrated p.
    silver-point p.
    smooth p.
    soldering p.
    Steiglitz p.
    stretching p.
    Tweed p.

P-50 light cured res·in bond·ed
ce·ram·ic

PLLA
    poly (L-lactic acid)

plug·ger
    amalgam p.
    automatic p.
    back-action p.
    endodontic p.
    finger p.
    foil p.
    foot p.
    gold p.
    Ladamore p.
    reverse p.
    root canal p.

plug·ger-spread·er

Plum·mer
    P.-Vinson syndrome

PMA in·dex

PME abut·ment

PMMA
polymethyl methacrylate

PMMA ce·ment

pneu·mo·ceph·a·lus

pock·et
absolute p.
complex p.
compound p.
gingival p.
infrabony p.
intra-alveolar p.
intrabony p.
periodontal p.
pyorrhea p.
relative p.
simple p.
subcrestal p.
suprabony p.
supracrestal p.

po·go·ni·on

point
p. A
abrasive p.
p. of an abscess
absorbent p.
acupuncture p.
alveolar p.
p. angle
p. ANS
p. Ar
auricular p.
p. B
p. Ba
p. ba
Barker's p.
p. bb
bilateral p.
p. Bo
boiling p.
boiling p., normal
Bolton p.
bony p.

point *(continued)*
bony end p.
Brinell hardness indenter
p.
Brinell indenter p.
Broadbent registration p.
Broca's p.
carborundum p.
central-bearing p.
Ceramisté p.
p. centric
cold rigor p.
condenser p.
condylar p.
contact p.
convenience p.
craniometric p.
critical p.
p. defect
diamond p.
p's douloureux
p. of election
end p.
equivalence p.
eye p.
freezing p.
gingival p.
p. Gl
p. Gn
p. Go
gutta-percha p.
hardness indenter p.
hinge-axis p.
Hirschfeld's silver p.
p. Id
p. IdI
p. IdS
immunodominant p.
indenter p.
p. Is
isoelectric p.
isoionic p.
jugal p.
jugomaxillary p.
Knoop hardness indenter
p.
Knoop indenter p.
p. KR

point *(continued)*
    lacrimal p.
    leak p.
    p. Li
    p. Ls
    M p.
    McEwen's p.
    maximum occipital p.
    p. Me
    median mandibular p.
    melting p.
    mental p.
    metopic p.
    midsagittal p.
    motor p.
    mounted p.
    mounted touch-up p.
    p. Na
    nasal p.
    normal boiling p.
    p. Ns
    occipital p.
    p. Or
    paper p.
    p. PNS
    p. Po.
    p. Pog
    polishing p.
    pour p.
    p. Pr
    preauricular p.
    pressure p.
    p. Ptm
    p. R
    Rockwell hardness
      indenter p.
    Rockwell indenter p.
    root canal p.
    rotary mounted p.
    p. S
    p. Sa
    p. SE
    p. Si
    silver p's
    p. Sn
    p. SO
    soft tissue p.
    p. S. Or

point *(continued)*
    p. Sp
    p. Sph
    spinal p.
    p. St
    starting p.
    subnasal p.
    subtemporal p.
    supra-auricular p.
    supra-articular p.
    supranasal p.
    sylvian p.
    p. Tr
    Vickers hardness indenter
      p.
    Vickers indenter p.
    Vogt's p.
    Vogt-Hueter p.
    white p.
    wood p.
    p. Z
    p. Zy

point·ing

Poi·ri·er
    P's line

poi·son·ing
    heavy metal p.

po·lar·i·scope
    circular p.

pol·ish
    Acrilustre P.

pol·ish·ing
    p. brush
    electro-p.
    metallographic p.
    p. of occlusion

Po·lo·caine

poly·cy·the·mia
    p. vera

poly·dac·ty·ly
    short rib–p., Majewski
      type

poly·dac·ty·ly *(continued)*
    short rib–p., non-Majewski
      type

poly·di·ox·an·one

poly·es·ter

poly·ether

poly·eth·y·lene

poly·glac·tin

Poly·jel NF im·pres·sion ma·
te·ri·al

poly·lac·tic acid

poly-L-lac·tic acid

poly-L-lac·tide

poly·mer
    cold-cured p's
    condensation p.
    cross-linked p.
    HTR p.
    thermoplastic p.
    thermosetting p.

poly·mer·ic

poly·mer·iza·tion
    addition p.
    condensation p.

poly·meth·acry·late

poly·meth·yl
    p. methacrylate (PMMA)

poly·mor·phous

poly·os·tot·ic

pol·yp
    fibroepithelial p.

poly·pro·py·lene

poly·sil·ox·ane
    vinyl p.

poly·sil·ox·ane/sil·i·cone

poly·sty·rene

poly·sul·fide

poly·sul·fone

poly·tet·ra·flu·o·ro·eth·y·lene
    p.-aluminum oxide
    p.-carbon
    Teflon p. (PTFE)

poly·ure·thane

Poly-Vi-Flor

poly·vi·nyl
    p. acetate
    p. chloride

poly·vi·nyl·ac·e·tate

poly·vi·nyl al·co·hol

poly·vi·nyl·ben·zene

poly·vi·nyl·chlo·ride

poly·vi·nyl·sil·ox·ane

Pont
    P. index

pon·tic
    porcelain-fused-to-metal
     (PFM) p's

por·ce·lain
    aluminous p.
    Ames plastic p.
    Biobond p.
    body shade p's
    p. cement
    Ceramco II p.
    dental p.
    high fusing p.
    high temperature
     maturing p.
    Jenkins' p.
    low-fusing p.
    low temperature maturing
     p.
    medium-fusing p.
    medium temperature
     maturing p.
    opaque p.
    Spectrum p.
    S.S. White new filling p.
    synthetic p.

Por·ce·lain Etch

por·ce·la·ne·ous

Por·ce·lite ce·ment

po·ri·on

po·ros·i·ty
    back pressure p.
    occluded gas p.
    shrink-spot p.
    solidification p.

por·phy·ria

porte·pol·ish·er
    contra-angle p.

po·si·tion
    centric p.
    condylar hinge p.
    distoangular p.
    eccentric p.
    eccentric test p's
    hinge p.
    hinge p., condylar
    hinge p., mandibular
    hinge p., terminal
    horizontal p.
    lateral occlusal p.
    mandibular hinge p.
    median occlusal p.
    occlusal p.
    occlusal retrusive p.
    physiologic rest p.
    posterior border p.
    protrusive occlusal p.
    rest p.
    terminal hinge p.
    tooth p.

po·si·tion·er
    tooth p.

post
    abutment p.
    Dentatus anchorage p.
    dowel p.
    implant p.
    P.W. (Pullen-Warner) split
      p.

post *(continued)*
    screw p.

post·con·den·sa·tion

pos·tero·clu·sion

po·tas·si·um
    p. fluoride

po·ten·tial
    bioelectric p.

Potts
    P. cross bar elevator
    P. elevator
    P. root pick

pouch
    snuff p.

pow·der
    Plastodent elastic
      impression p.
    zinc oxide p.

Pow·er Bond bond·ing sys·tem

Pra·der
    P.-Willi syndrome

pre·ce·men·tum

Pre·cise im·pres·sion ma·te·ri·al

pre·den·tin

Pre·dent top·i·cal flu·o·ride
    treat·ment gel

pred·nis·o·lone

pre·go·ni·um

Pre·line base/lin·er

pre·max·il·lary

pre·mo·lar
    first p.

pre·odon·to·blast

prep
    Enamel Etchant enamel p.

prep·a·ra·tion
    apical p.
    biomechanical p.
    cavity p.

pre·pros·thet·ic

pre·pu·ber·tal

Pres·i·dent im·pres·sion ma·
    te·ri·al

P-10 res·in bond·ed ce·ram·ic
    com·pos·ite

Pres·so·mat·ic at·tach·ment

Pres·so·mat·ic unit

pres·sure
    biting p.
    lip p.
    occlusal p.

Pre·ven·tion mouth·rinse

Pre·vox pick·ling so·lu·tion

Prich·ard
    P. curet
    P. periosteal elevator

prim·er
    cavity p.

pri·mor·di·al

prin·ci·ple
    bone induction p.

prism
    adamantine p's
    enamel p's

Pris·ma AP.H com·pos·ite res·
    in

Pris·ma AP.H re·stor·a·tive

Pris·ma Opa·quers

Pris·ma-Shield pit and fis·sure
    seal·ant

Pris·ma Tints

Pris·ma Uni·ver·sal Bond
    bond·ing sys·tem

Pris·ma Uni·ver·sal Bond 2
    bond·ing sys·tem

Pris·ma Uni·ver·sal Bond 3
    bond·ing sys·tem

Pris·ma VLC Dy·cal cal·ci·um
    hy·drox·ide base

probe
    Bowman's p.
    Brackett's p's
    calibrated p.
    CPITN-E p.
    cross p.
    Expros explorer/p.
    Fox-Williams p.
    Glickman p.
    Goldman-Fox p.
    Marquis p.
    Michigan p.
    Michigan "O" round p.
    Nabers p.
    perio p.
    periodontal p.
    pocket p.
    root canal p.
    Williams p.
    Williams' periodontal p.
    Williams Round p.

Pro·caine

Pro-Care flu·o·ride so·lu·tion

Pro-Care Pro·phy paste

pro·ce·dure
    Brosch p.
    Edlan-Mejchar p.
    Kole p.
    lysis p.
    Millard p.
    Sistrunk p.
    von Langenbeck p.
    W-plasty p.

pro·cess
    alveolar p.
    coronoid p.
    dental p.
    mental p.

pro·cess *(continued)*
    p. of odontoblast
    odontoblastic p.
    temporal p. of mandible
    Tomes p.

pro·ces·sus *pl.* pro·ces·sus
    p. retromandibularis
        glandulae parotidis

pro·col·la·gen

Pro·co·Sol seal·er

Prof·fit
    Ackerman-P. classification
        (for malocclusion)

pro·file
    concave p.
    convex p.

Pro·Flex im·pres·sion ma·te·ri·al

Pro·flex scal·ers

Pro·flex scal·ing strip

pro·ge·nia

prog·na·thia

prog·na·thic

prog·na·thism
    mandibular p.
    maxillary p.

prog·na·thom·e·ter

prog·na·thous

pro·jec·tion
    bregma-mentum p.
    enamel p's
    extradental p.
    lateral jaw p.
    lateral oblique p. of
        mandible
    mental p.
    submentovertex p.

Pro·lene suture

pro·lif·er·a·tive

prop
    mouth p.

pro·phy·lax·is
    dental p.
    oral p.

Pro·phy Prep den·tal stain re·mov·er

Pro·pi·on·i·bac·te·ri·um
    P. acnes

Pro·plast

Pro·plast-Tef·lon TMJ im·plant

pro·por·tion
    facial p's
    vertical facial p.

pro·pul·sor

Pro Sol CHX ir·ri·gat·ing so·lu·tion

pros·ta·glan·din
    p. $F_{2\alpha}$
    p. $F_{2\alpha}$tromethamine

pros·the·sis *pl.* pros·the·ses
    AO/ASIF condylar
        prostheses
    cleft palate p.
    complete dental p.
    condylar p.
    dental p.
    fixed p.
    fixed bridge p.
    Fossa-Eminence p.
    implant-supported
        prostheses
    maxillary p.
    maxillofacial p.
    mouthstick p.
    obturator p.
    overlay p.
    partial denture p.
    permanent p.
    speech-aid p.
    swinglock p.
    telescopic p.

pros·the·sis *(continued)*
    temporary p.
    TMJ Condylar P.
    TMJ Fossa Eminence P.

pros·thet·ic

pros·thet·ics
    complete denture p.
    dental p.
    denture p.
    facial p.
    full denture p.
    maxillofacial p.

pros·tho·don·tia

pros·tho·don·tics
    complete p.
    crown and bridge p.
    fixed p.
    fixed bridge p.
    maxillofacial p.
    partial p.
    removable p.
    removable partial p.

pros·tho·don·tist

pro·ta·form

pro·tec·tor
    Dentin P.

pro·tein
    bone morphogenetic p.
    (BMP)
    C-reactive p.
    S-100 p.

pro·tein·o·sis
    lipoid p.

Pro-Temp crown and bridge
ma·te·ri·al

Pro·te·us
    P. mirabilis
    P. vulgaris

Pro·tex·in Oral Rinse

pro·to·cone

pro·to·co·nid

pro·trac·tion
    mandibular p.
    maxillary p.

pro·tru·sion
    bimaxillary p.
    bimaxillary dentoalveolar
      p.
    double p.
    forward p.
    jaw p.
    lateral p.
    mandibular p.
    maxillary p.
    maxillary alveolar p.

pro·tu·ber·ance
    p. of chin

pro·tru·sion
    bimaxillary dentoalveolar
      p.

Pro·vis·cell ce·ment

Prox·i·gel oral an·ti·sep·tic
cleans·er

prox·i·mo·buc·cal

prox·i·mo·la·bi·al

prox·i·mo·lin·gual

pseu·do·an·eu·rysm

pseu·do·ar·thro·sis

pseu·do·cyst
    p. of maxillary sinus

pseu·do·gout

pseu·do·hy·po·para·
thy·roi·dism

Pseu·do·mo·nas
    P. aeruginosa

pseu·do·os·teo·ar·thri·tis

pseu·do·prog·na·thism

pso·ri·a·sis

PTFE
    polytetrafluoroethylene

P.T. pulp treat·ment

pty·a·lec·ta·sis

pty·a·lize

pty·a·lo·li·thot·o·my

P-type ream·er

pulp
    coronal p.
    dead p.
    p. death
    dental p.
    devitalized p.
    enamel p.
    exposed p.
    mummified p.
    p. necrosis
    necrotic p.
    nonvital p.
    putrescent p.
    radicular p.
    tooth p.
    vital p.

pul·pal·gia
    acute p.
    advanced acute p.
    chronic p.
    hyperactive p.
    hypersensitive p.
    incipient acute p.
    moderate acute p.
    severe acute p.

Pulp·dent li·quid

Pulp·dent pulp cap·ping agent

Pulp·dent sy·ringe

pul·pec·to·my

pul·pit·i·des

pul·pi·tis *pl.* pul·pit·i·des
    acute p.
    anachoretic p.
    p. aperta
    chronic p.
    chronic hyperplastic p.
    p. clausa

pul·pi·tis *(continued)*
    closed p.
    generalized p.
    hyperplastic p.
    hypertrophic p.
    irreversible p.
    open p.
    partial p.
    reversible p.
    suppurative p.
    total p.

pulp·less

pul·pot·o·my
    cervical p.

pu·mex

pum·ice

punch
    pin p.
    plate p.
    rubber dam p.

pur·pu·ra
    idiopathic
        thrombocytopenic p.

push·er
    band p.

put·ty
    CutterSil P.
    Reprosil Quixx P.

P.W. (Pullen-Warner) bolt

P.W. (Pullen-Warner) split post

pyk·no·dys·os·to·sis

Pyle
    P. metaphyseal dysplasia

pyo·gen·ic

py·or·rhea
    p. alveolaris
    schmutz p.

py·or·rhe·al

pyo·sto·ma·ti·tis
    p. vegetans

Py·rex glass

py·ru·vate

quad·ran·gle

quad·ran·gu·lar

quad·rant

quad·ri·cus·pid

Qua·tre·fage
   Q's angle

Quin·by
   Q. scissors

quin·o·lones

quin·que·cus·pid

R
Broadbent registration
point
right

Ra·cer
R. handpiece

Ra·cord re·trac·tion cord

ra·dec·to·my

ra·di·a·tion
electron beam r.

ra·di·ec·to·my

ra·dio·graph
bite-wing r.
cephalometric r.
extraoral r.
interproximal r.
intraoral r.
occlusal r.
panoramic r.
periapical r.

ra·dio·graph·ic

ra·di·og·ra·phy
panoramic r.

ra·dio·lu·cent

ra·di·sec·to·my

Ra·dix An·chor sys·tem

Ram·fjord
R. index

Ra·mi·tec bite reg·is·tra·tion ma·te·ri·al

ramp
bite r's

ra·mus *pl.* ra·mi
rami dentales arteriae
alveolaris inferioris

ra·mus *(continued)*
rami dentales arteriarum
alveolarium superiorum
anteriorum
rami dentales arteriae
alveolaris superioris
posterioris
rami dentales inferiores
plexus dentalis inferioris
rami dentales superiores
plexus dentalis superioris
r. of jaw
rami linguales nervi
glossopharyngei
rami linguales nervi
hypoglossi
rami linguales nervi
lingualis
r. of mandible
r. mandibulae

Ranke
R's angle

ran·u·la
plunging r.

Rapp
R.-Hodgkin ectodermal
dysplasia syndrome

RA-2 ramus frame implants

Rasch·kow
plexus of R.

rash
wandering r.

rasp
bone r.

rate
DEF (decayed, extracted,
and filled) r.
DMF (decayed, missing,
and filled) r.
periodontal disease r.

ra·tio
    alloy-mercury r.
    crown-root r.
    holdaway r.
    W/P (water-powder) r.

RAU
    recurrent aphthous ulcer

Ra·vo·caine

RC-Prep

RDA
    Registered Dental
        Assistant

RDH
    Registered Dental
        Hygienist

re·ac·tion
    cinnamon r.
    drug r's
    foreign body r.
    Mazotti r.
    mouthwash r's
    toothpaste r's

ream·er
    A-type r.
    B-1 r.
    B-2 r.
    D-type r.
    engine r.
    FilLock r.
    Flexi-Post r.
    Giro engine r's
    G-type r.
    Kerr r.
    Ko-type r.
    K-type r.
    M-type r.
    O-type r.
    Peeso r's
    P-type r.
    quarter-turn r.
    screw post r.
    T-type r.

re·at·tach·ment

re·base

re·bas·ing

re·bound
    gingival r.

re·cep·to·ma
    fibronectin-integrin r.

re·ces·sion
    bone r.
    gingival r.
    index gingival r.
    pathologic r.

re·cip·ro·ca·tion
    active r.
    passive r.

re·con·struc·tion
    condylar r.
    maxillary r.

Re·con tis·sue con·di·tion·er
    and func·tion·al im·pres·
    sion ma·te·ri·al

re·con·tour

rec·ord
    centric interocclusal r.
    centric maxillomandibular
        r.
    centric occluding relation r.
    chew-in r., functional
    dental r.
    eccentric r.
    eccentric interocclusal r.
    eccentric
        maxillomandibular r.
    face-bow r.
    functional chew-in r.
    insurance summary r.
    interocclusal r.
    interocclusal r., centric
    interocclusal r., eccentric
    interocclusal r., lateral
    interocclusal r., protrusive
    jaw relation r.
    lateral check-bite
        interocclusal r.

rec·ord *(continued)*
    lateral interocclusal r.
    maxillomandibular r.
    occluding centric relation r.
    Opotow jaw relation r's
    profile r.
    protrusive r.
    protrusive interocclusal r.
    terminal jaw relation r.
    3-D (three-dimensional) r.
    three-dimensional r.

re·cov·ery

re·cry·stal·li·za·tion

Red Cote dis·clos·ing tab·lets

Red·phase-P

re·duc·tion
    chin r.
    closed r.
    malar r.
    open r.

re·flec·tor
    dental r.

re·flex
    gag r.
    pharyngeal r.

re·gain·er
    space r.
    split acrylic spring spacer
      r.
    spring spacer r.

re·gain·er-main·tain·er
    jackscrew r.-m.

re·gen·er·a·tion
    condylar r.
    guided tissue r.

re·gion
    mylohyoid r.

re·gion·al

Re·gi·sil bite reg·is·tra·tion
ma·te·ri·al

Reg·is·tered Den·tal Hy·gien·
ist (RDH)

reg·is·tra·tion
    bite r.
    functional occlusal r.
    maxillomandibular r.
    tissue r.

Reg·no·li
    R's operation

re·im·plan·ta·tion

Rei·ter
    R's syndrome

re·la·tion
    acentric r.
    acquired eccentric jaw r.
    buccolingual r.
    centric r.
    centric jaw r.
    convenience jaw r.
    cusp-fossa r.
    dynamic r's
    eccentric r.
    eccentric jaw r.
    eccentric jaw r., acquired
    intermaxillary r.
    jaw r.
    lateral occlusal r.
    maxillomandibular r.
    median r.
    median jaw r.
    median occlusal r.
    median retruded jaw r.
    occluding r.
    occlusal r.
    posterior border jaw r.
    protrusive jaw r.
    rest r.
    rest jaw r.
    retruded jaw r.
    ridge r.
    static r's
    surgical jaw r.
    unstrained jaw r.
    working bite r.

re·la·tion·ship
 buccolingual r.
 transverse r.

re·lief
 gingival r.

re·line
 denture r.
 Hydrocryl denture r.
 Kooliner denture r.
 LiteLine dental r.
 Molloplast-B denture r.
 Softline denture r.
 Tru-Soft denture r.
 Truliner denture r.

re·lin·er
 Just Treatment r.

re·lin·ing
 denture r.

re·mod·el·ing
 osteoclastic r.

re·mov·er
 band r.
 crown r.
 crown and bridge r.
 Prophy Prep dental stain r.

re·pair
 histologic tooth r.
 periapical tooth r.
 radiographic tooth r.

re·plan·ta·tion

re·po·si·tion·ing
 jaw r.

Rep·ro·sil im·pres·sion ma·te·ri·al

Rep·ro·sil Quixx put·ty

re·sec·tion
 maxillary r.
 root r.

re·shap·ing
 occlusal r.

re·sid·u·al

re·sil·i·ence

re·sil·i·en·cy

Re·si·lute

Re·si·ment ce·ment

res·in
 acrylic r's
 activated r.
 Adaptic II composite r.
 AH26 r.
 Alike r.
 alkyd r.
 autopolymer r.
 r. benjamin
 r. benzoin
 Bisfil I composite r.
 r. cement
 Coe Ortho r.
 cold-curing r.
 composite r.
 Concise White Sealant r.
 copolymer r.
 crazing r.
 crown and bridge r.
 cyanoacrylate r.
 dammar r.
 dental r.
 denture base r.
 direct filling r.
 Distalite composite r.
 Duralay inlay r.
 epoxy r.
 Estilux Posterior
  composite r.
 Fermit composite r.
 Fiber-Pink acrylic r.
 Fiber-Pink Triad r.
 filled r.
 r. filler
 free particle composite r.
 Ful-Fil composite r.
 heat polymerized r.
 heat-curing r.
 Heliomolar r.
 Heliomolar composite r.
 HelioProgress r.

res·in *(continued)*
    Herculite Condensable
      composite r.
    Herculite XRV composite r.
    ionomer r.
    kauri r.
    Lucitone 199 denture base
      r.
    r. matrix
    microfil r.
    4-META adhesive r.
    microfilled composite r.
    natural r.
    Nuva-PA composite r.
    Paragon acrylic r.
    Pattern acrylic r.
    P-10 composite r.
    P-30 composite r.
    Perfex repair r.
    photoelastic r.
    polycarbonate r.
    polyurethane r.
    Prisma AP.H composite r.
    quick-cure r.
    repair r.
    restorative r.
    self-curing r.
    Sinter-Fil II composite r.
    Status composite r.
    styrene r.
    Super Soft soft acrylic r.
    synthetic r.
    thermoset r.
    thermosetting r.
    thermosetting
      methacrylate r.
    Tytin composite r.
    ultraviolet light-cured r.
    unfilled r.
    urethane dimethacrylate r.
    urethane-modified bis-
      GMA composite r.
    vinyl r.
    visible light–cured r.
    Visio-Fil composite r.
    yellow r.

re·sis·tant

re·sorp·tion
    apical r.
    apical root r.
    bone r.
    cementum r.
    central r.
    cervical r.
    condylar r.
    external r.
    external root r.
    external tooth r.
    extracanalicular r.
    frontal r.
    gingival r.
    horizontal r.
    idiopathic r.
    internal r.
    internal tooth r.
    intracanalicular r.
    lateral r.
    osteoclastic r.
    physiologic r.
    rear r.
    root r.
    surface root r.
    tooth r.
    undermining r.
    unerupted tooth r.
    vertical r.

rest
    r. area
    auxiliary implant r.
    auxiliary occlusal r.
    cingulum r.
    continuous bar r.
    finger r.
    incisal r.
    internal r.
    intracoronal r.
    lingual r.
    Malassez r.
    nasal r.
    occlusal r.
    precision r.
    recessed r.
    root r.
    semiprecision r.

rest *(continued)*
    surface r.

rest·bite

res·to·ra·tion
    alloy r.
    buccal r.
    composite r.
    cusp r.
    direct gold r.
    distal extension r.
    facial r.
    implant r.
    intermediate r.
    metal-ceramic r.
    overlay r.
    permanent r.
    pin-supported r.
    porcelain-bonded r.
    porcelain fused to metal r.
    prosthetic r.
    temporary r.
    r. of vertical dimension

re·stor·a·tive
    Adaptic dental r.
    Chelon-Silver glass
      ionomer r.
    Durafil r.
    EMKA r.
    EMKA-Fil glass ionomer
      dental r.
    Finesse r.
    Fuji II r.
    Fuji Cap II r.
    Fuji II glass ionomer r.
    Fuji II LC glass ionomer r.
    Ful-Fil r.
    ionomer r.
    IRM r.
    Ketac-Fil r.
    Ketac-Silver glass ionomer/
      silver r.
    Miracle Mix r.
    Prisma AP.H r.
    Silux Plus r.
    Silux Plus L.C. r.
    Sun-Schein r.

re·stor·a·tive *(continued)*
    Visio-Dispers r.
    Visio-Fil r.
    Z100 r.

Re·stor·il

re·tain·er
    band and spur r.
    continuous r.
    continuous bar r.
    coping r.
    direct r.
    extracoronal r.
    fixed r.
    Hawley r.
    I-bar r's
    indirect r.
    intracoronal r.
    lingual r.
    matrix r.
    multiple r's
    precision r.
    screw r.
    secondary r.
    space r.
    Tach-E-Z r.

re·tard·er
    gypsum r.

re·ten·tion
    r. area of tooth
    r. arm
    clip r.
    denture r.
    direct r.
    extracoron r.
    frictional wall r.
    indirect r.
    intracoronal-extracoronal
      r.
    partial denture r.
    surgical r.

re·tic·u·lo·en·do·the·li·o·sis
    lipid r.

re·tic·u·lo·sis
    lethal midline r.
    midline malignant r.

re·tic·u·lo·sis *(continued)*
    polymorphic r.

re·tic·u·lum *pl.* re·tic·u·la
    stellate r.

re·trac·tion
    gingival r.
    mandibular r.

re·trac·tor
    Austin r.
    beaver-tail r.
    Bishop r.
    Black r.
    Brinker tissue r.
    cat's-paw r.
    cheek and lip r.
    cheek and tongue r.
    Columbia r.
    Henahan r.
    Le Vasseur-Merrill r.
    lip r.
    Minnesota r.
    Moorehead's r.
    Nu-Lite r.
    Obwegeser ramus r.
    rake r.
    ribbon r.
    Seldin r.
    Senn r.
    Shuman r.
    University of Minnesota r.
    vein hook r.
    Wieder r.

Re·trax re·trac·tion cord

Re·treat re·trac·tion cord

Re·treat II re·trac·tion cord

re·triev·er
    Caulfield r.
    lasso-type suture r.
    silver-point r.

ret·ro·dis·cal

ret·ro·fill·ing

ret·ro·gna·thia

ret·ro·gnath·ic

ret·ro·gnath·ism
    mandibular r.

ret·ro·vi·rus

re·tru·sion
    mandibular r.
    maxillary r.

Ret·zi·us
    R's line
    R. parallel stria
    stripe of R.

Re·veal dis·clos·ing so·lu·tion

Re·veal dis·clos·ing tab·lets

Rey·nolds
    R. pliers

R for·ceps

rhab·do·my·o·ma

rhab·do·myo·sar·co·ma

rhi·zo·don·tro·py

rhi·zo·don·try·py

RHN
    Rockwell hardness number

Rhodes
    R. back-action chisel

Rich·ards
    R. screws

Rich·ey
    R. condyle marker

Rich·mond
    R. crown

rick·ets
    pseudo–vitamin D
        deficiency r.
    vitamin D–resistant r.
    X-linked
        hypophosphatemic r.

ridge
    alveolar r.

ridge *(continued)*
    alveolar r., residual
    basal r.
    buccocervical r.
    buccogingival r.
    dental r.
    edentulous r's
    incisal r.
    linguocervical r.
    linguogingival r.
    longitudinal r. of hard
      palate
    r. of mandibular neck
    marginal r.
    mylohyoid r.
    oblique r.
    palatine r's, transverse
    pterygoid r.
    residual r.
    transverse r.
    triangular r.

Rie·ger
    R's syndrome

RIF
    rigid internal fixation

Riggs
    R. disease

rim
    bite r.
    occlusion r.
    record r.

Rim-Lock im·pres·sion tray

Ring
    Hade-R. attachment

ring
    casting r.
    neonatal r.

rinse
    chlorhexidine r.
    mouth r's
    Plax dental r.
    Protexin Oral R.

Ris·don
    R. approach
    R. incision
    R's wire

RITE
    rapid intraoperative tissue
      expander

Rite Bite tray

Rit·ter
    R. tester

Riv·et
    R's angle

Ri·vi·nus
    canal of R.
    duct of R.
    R. gland

RME
    rapid maxillary expansion

Roach
    R. attachment
    R. carver
    R. clasp

Rob·ert
    R. wiring

Rob·erts
    R.-SC phocomelia
      syndrome

Ro·bin
    R. sequence

Ro·bi·now
    R's syndrome

Ro·ches·ter
    R.-Péan hemostat

Rock·well
    R. hardness indenter point
    R. hardness number
      (RHN)
    R. hardness scale
    R. hardness test
    R. indenter

Rock·well *(continued)*
> R. indenter point
> R. scale

rod
> ear r's
> enamel r's

Rog·er An·der·son
> R.A. pin

roll
> braided cotton r's

ron·geur
> Blumenthal r.
> mini-Friedman r.

root
> accessory r's
> anatomical r.
> lingual r.
> palatine r.
> physiological r.
> retained r.
> r. of tongue
> r. of tooth

Ro·sen·thal
> Melkersson-R. syndrome

ro·sette
> strain gauge r.

ro·sin

Ross
> R. tissue scissors

Ro·ta-dent plaque re·mov·al de·vice

ro·ta·tion

Roth·er·mann
> R. attachment

Roth·mund
> R.-Thomson syndrome

Ro·to-Pro scal·er

rouge
> green r.
> jeweler's r.

Rowe
> R. maxillary disimpaction forceps
> R. zygomatic awl
> R. zygomatic elevator

Roy·al al·loy

RPC
> recurrent parotitis in childhood

RPD
> removable partial denture

RPE
> rapid palatal expansion

RP-I bar

RTV
> room temperature vulcanization

RTV sil·i·cone

rub·ber
> r. dam
> silicone r.
> SIR silicone impression r.

Rub·ber·loid im·pres·sion ma·te·ri·al

ru·bel·la

ru·be·o·la

Ru·bin·stein
> R.-Taybi syndrome

Ruf·fi·ni
> R. endings

ru·ga *pl.* ru·gae
> rugae palatinae
> palatine rugae

rule
> buccal object r.
> Clark's r.

Rus·sell
    R. index
    R.-Silver syndrome

Ru·val·ca·ba
    R's syndrome

Ry·der
    R. needle holder

sac
  dental s.
  enamel s.

sac·cu·lus *pl.* sac·cu·li
  s. dentis

sad·dle
  denture base s.

Sae·thre
  S.-Chotzen syndrome

sag
  condylar s.

sa·li·va
  chorda s.
  ganglionic s.
  lingual s.
  parotid s.
  ropy s.
  sublingual s.
  submaxillary s.
  sympathetic s.

sal·i·vant

sal·i·vary

sal·i·vate

sal·i·va·tion

sal·i·va·to·ry

Sal·ter
  S's line

Salz·burg ti·ta·ni·um plat·ing sys·tem

San·fi·lip·po
  S's syndrome

San·to·ri·ni
  S's muscle

Sap·pey
  S's ligament

sar·coid

sar·co·ma *pl.* sar·co·mas, sar·co·ma·ta
  epithelioid s.
  Ewing's s.
  fasciculated s.
  granulocytic s.
  high-grade surface s.
  juxtacortical s.
  Kaposi's s.
  multicentric osteogenic s.
  nerve sheath s.
  neurogenic s.
  neurogenous s.
  osteogenic s.
  parosteal osteogenic s.
  periosteal osteogenic s.
  peripheral nerve s.
  soft-tissue osteogenic s.
  synovial s.
  telangiectatic osteogenic s.

Sas·sou·ni
  S. analysis

saw
  Horico Ribbon S.
  Joseph's s.
  Koeber's s.
  separating s.

scale
  Abbreviated Injury S.
  Brinell s.
  Brinell hardness s.
  Knoop s.
  Knoop hardness s.
  Mohs s.
  Mohs hardness s.
  Rockwell s.
  Rockwell hardness s.
  Vickers s.
  Vickers hardness s.

sca·ler
  Cattoni s.
  chisel s.

sca·ler *(continued)*
    Crane Kaplan s.
    Darby-Perry s.
    deep s.
    double-ended s.
    Goldman-Fox s.
    hoe s.
    Jaquette s.
    Kirkland s.
    McCall s.
    Orban hoe s.
    Proflex s.
    Roto-Pro s's
    sickle s.
    superficial s.
    Taylor s.
    Towner s.
    ultrasonic s.
    Whiteside s.
    wing s.
    Younger s.
    Younger Good s.

scal·ing
    coronal s.
    deep s.
    hand s.
    root s.
    rotary s.
    subgingival s.
    supragingival s.
    ultrasonic s.

scapho·ceph·a·ly

scar
    periapical s.

scar·let fe·ver

Schatz·mann
    S. attachment

Scheie
    Hurler-S. compound
        syndrome
    S's syndrome

Schin·zel
    S.-Giedion syndrome

Schir·mer
    S. test

Schlug·er
    S. file

Schmecke·bier
    S. apexo elevator

Schreg·er
    line of S.
    S's stria
    zone of S.

Schu·big·er
    S. attachment

Schül·ler
    Hand-Christian-S.
        syndrome
    Hand-S.-Christian disease
    S's disease

Schwann
    S. cell

schwan·no·ma
    malignant s.
    malignant s. of the palate
    metaplastic malignant s.

schwan·no·sar·co·ma

Schwartz
    S.-Jampel syndrome

Schwarz
    S. activator
    S. appliance
    S. classification (of
        orthodontic forces)

sci·ence
    materials s.

scin·tig·ra·phy
    parotid s.
    sequential quantitative s.
    technetium 99m s.

scis·sel

scis·sors
    angled s.
    crown and collar s.

scis·sors *(continued)*
    Dean s.
    Fox s.
    Glickman s.
    Goldman-Fox s.
    Hu-Friedy s.
    Kelly s.
    Lagrange's s.
    Lister s.
    Liston's s.
    Littauer s.
    Mayo s.
    northbent s.
    operating s.
    Quinby s.
    Ross tissue s.
    Spencer s.
    straight s.
    Sullivan s.
    surgical s.
    suture s.
    tissue s.
    Wagner s.

scis·sors-bite

SCLE
    subacute lupus
      erythematosus

scle·ro·der·ma

scle·rom·e·ter

scle·ro·scope

scle·ros·ing

scle·ro·sis
    amyotrophic lateral s.
    progressive systemic s.
    tuberous s.

scle·ros·te·o·sis

score
    oral hygiene s.
    periodontal s.
    periodontal disease s.

Scotch·bond bond·ing sys·tem

Scotch·bond 2 bond·ing sys·tem

Scotch·bond den·tal ad·he·sive

Scotch·bond etch·ing gel

Scott
    S. attachment

scrap·er
    Vul-Crylic s.

screen
    oral s.
    vestibular s.

screw
    adjustable s.
    AO s.
    bicortical s.
    bicortical compression lag
      s's
    bicortical position s's
    bone s.
    Carroll-Girard s.
    coping s.
    cortex s.
    cortical s.
    emergency s's
    expansion s.
    implant s.
    lag s.
    orthodontic s.
    orthodontic expansion s.
    osteosynthesis s's
    ovalhead-crossdrive s.
    pretapped s's
    pull s.
    Richards s's
    self-tapping s's
    TiMesh bone s's
    titanium s's
    Wurzburg s's

screw-post

Screw-Vent im·plant

scrof·u·la

S-C zinc phos·phate ce·ment

seal
    border s.
    cavity s.

seal *(continued)*
- double s.
- hermetic s.
- palatal s.
- posterior palatal s.
- postpalatal s.

seal·ant
- Barrier dentin s.
- Concise s.
- Concise Light Cured White S.
- contact dentin s.
- Defender pit and fissure s.
- Delton pit and fissure s.
- dental s.
- fibrin s.
- fissure s.
- Fluoroshield pit and fissure s.
- Helioseal pit and fissure s.
- pit and fissure s.
- Prisma-Shield pit and fissure s.
- Seal-Rite pit and fissure s.
- Visio-Seal pit and fissure s.

Seal·apex root ca·nal seal·er

seal·er
- calciobiotic root canal s.
- endodontic s.
- Kerr S.
- Ketac glass-ionomer s.
- NOgenol root canal s.
- ProcoSol s.
- root canal s.
- Sealapex root canal s.

Seal-Rite pit and fis·sure seal·ant

seat
- basal s.
- rest s.

seat·er
- band s.

se·ba·ceous

Se·bi·leau
- S's hollow

seb·or·rhe·ic

Seck·el
- S. syndrome

se·co·dont

Se·co·nal

se·cre·tion
- antilytic s.

sec·to·ri·al

se·da·tion
- intravenous s.
- oral s.

Sel·din
- S. elevator
- S. periosteal elevator
- S. retractor
- S. straight elevator

se·lec·tion
- shade s.
- tooth s.
- tooth color s.

se·le·no·dont

Se·le·no·mo·nas
- *S. sputigena*

Sem·ken
- S.-Taylor forceps

se·nes·cence
- dental s.

Senn
- S. retractor

sen·si·tiv·i·ty
- tooth s.
- s. to percussion
- s. to tactile stimulation
- s. to temperature changes

Sen·ter
- S. syndrome

sep·a·ra·tion
    gradual tooth s.
    immediate tooth s.
    mechanical s.
    slow tooth s.
    tooth s.

sep·a·ra·tor
    elastomeric s.
    Ferrier's s.
    True's s.

se·pi·um

sep·to·plas·ty

sep·tum *pl.* sep·ta
    s. alveoli
    gingival s.
    gum s.
    interalveolar s.
    interdental s.
    interradicular s.
    s. interradiculare
    s. intra-alveolarium

se·quence
    amyoplasia congenita
      disruptive s.
    anencephaly s.
    athyrotic hypothyroidism
      s.
    caudal dysplasia s.
    cleft lip s.
    DiGeorge s.
    early amnion rupture s.
    early amnion rupture s.
      (disruptive)
    frontonasal dysplasia s.
      (midline)
    holoprosencephaly s.
    Klippel-Feil s.
    linear sebaceous nevus s.
    Moebius s.
    Robin s.

Ser·ax

Ser·gen·ti paste

Ser·res
    S. angle

se·rum
    antilymphocyte s.

set·ting
    s. expansion
    s. time

set·up
    diagnostic s.

Sev·ri·ton cav·i·ty seal prim·
er

S file

shade
    Bioform body s's
    Ceramco body s's

shank
    bur s.

Shan·non
    S. drill

shap·ing
    root canal s.

sharp·en·er

Shar·pey
    S's fibers

Shea
    S.-Anthony antral balloon

shear

shears
    gauze s.

sheath
    dentinal s.
    enamel prism s.
    enamel rod s.
    epithelial root s.
    lingual s.
    prism s.
    rod s.
    root s.

Shel·don
    Freeman-S. syndrome

shelf
    buccal s.

shelf *(continued)*
    dental s.

shell
    acrylic resin s.

shel·lac

Sher·er
    S. attachment

Sher·man
    S. plate

shield
    buccal s.
    lingual s.
    lip s.
    oral s.

shift
    cone s.
    occlusal s.

shoe
    Neurohr-Williams s.
    Neurohr-Williams rest s.

shoe·ing
    s. cusp

Sho·fu spher·i·cal al·loy

Sho·fu Su·per Snap disk sys·tem

Sho·keir
    Pena-S. phenotype

shoul·der

Shprin·tzen
    S's syndrome

shrink·age
    casting s.
    s. compensation
    polymerization s.
    thermal s.

Shu·man
    S. retractor

si·al·a·den

si·al·ad·e·nec·to·my

si·al·ad·e·ni·tis
    s. papilliferum

si·al·ad·e·no·sis

si·al·ad·e·not·o·my

si·al·ec·ta·sia

si·al·ic

si·a·line

si·a·lo·ad·e·nec·to·my

si·a·lo·ad·e·not·o·my

si·alo·an·gi·ec·ta·sis

si·alo·do·cho·plas·ty

si·a·log·e·nous

si·a·log·ra·phy

si·alo·li·thi·a·sis

si·alo·li·thot·o·my

si·alo·meta·pla·sia
    necrotizing s.

si·a·lo-odon·to·gen·ic

si·a·lor·rhea

si·alo·sis

si·alo·sy·rinx

side
    balancing s.
    functioning s.
    nonfunctioning s.
    pressure s.
    safe s.
    tension s.
    working s.

sign
    Battle's s.
    Carabelli's s.
    Chvostek s.
    Verrill s.

Si·lain

Sil·a·mat me·chan·i·cal tri·tu·ra·tor

Sil·a·mat mix·ing unit

sil·ane
    hydrolyzed s.
    nonhydrolyzed s.
    preactivated s.

Si·las·tic 382

Si·las·tic 399

Si·las·tic 6508

Si·las·tic im·plant

Sil·ene sil·i·cone im·pres·sion ma·te·ri·al

si·lex

sil·i·ca

Sil·i·cap ce·ment

Sil·i·coat·er sil·i·ca coat·ing sys·tem

sil·i·coat·ing

sil·i·con
    s. carbide
    s. dioxide

sil·i·cone
    s. fluid
    s. putty
    room temperature-
        vulcanizing s.
    RTV (room
        temperature–vulcanizing)
        s.

Silky Rock den·tal stone

Sil-Trax re·trac·tion cord

Si·lux Plus L.C. re·stor·a·tive

Si·lux Plus re·stor·a·tive

Sil·ver
    Russell-S. syndrome

sil·ver
    s. nitrate

Sil·ver Crest al·loy

Sim·u·la·tor ad·just·able ar·tic·u·la·tor

Sim·ul·cure

sin·ter

Sin·ter-Fil II com·pos·ite res·in

si·nus *pl.* si·nus, si·nus·es
    cutaneous s.
    maxillary s.

si·nu·si·tis

SiO_2
    silicon dioxide

SIR im·pres·sion ma·te·ri·al

SIR sil·i·cone im·pres·sion rubber

Sir·is
    Coffin-S. syndrome

Sis·trunk
    S. procedure

60 Sec·ond Taste Flu·o·ride Gel

60:60 Rinse

Sjö·gren
    S's syndrome
    S.-Larsson syndrome

Skin·ner
    S's classification (for
        partially edentulous
        arches)

skull·cap

SLE
    systemic lupus
        erythematosus

sleeve
    precision-fitting s.

sling
    mandibular s.
    pterygomasseteric s.

slope
    basilar s.
    lower ridge s.
    mandibular
      anteroposterior ridge s.

slot
    bracket s.

Slu·der
    S's neuralgia

Smith
    Marshall-S. syndrome
    S's resin cement
    S's zinc cement
    S.-Lemli-Opitz syndrome

Snap crown and bridge ma·te·ri·al

Snap-Stone den·tal stone

snuff

so·cia
    s. parotidis

sock·et
    dry s.
    tooth s's

so·di·um
    s. fluoride

Sof-Lex con·tour·ing and pol·ish·ing discs

Sof-Lex fin·ish·ing and pol·ish·ing sys·tem

Sof-Lex Pop-On disk sys·tem

Sof-Lex Pop-On man·drel

So-Flo phos·phate top·i·cal gel

Sof·Scale cal·cu·lus scal·ing gel

Soft·line den·ture re·line

Sof·tone tis·sue con·di·tion·er and func·tion·al im·pres·sion ma·te·ri·al

sold·er
    building s.
    gold s.
    hard s.
    hardened s.
    silver s.
    soft s.
    softened s.
    sticky s.
    white s.

sol·der·ing

so·lu·tion
    benzocaine topical s.
    bleaching s.
    disclosing s.
    lidocaine hydrochloride oral topical s.
    lidocaine oral topical s.
    Nupro Neutral fluoride s.
    Prevox pickling s.
    Pro-Care fluoride s.
    Pro Sol CHX irrigating s.
    Reveal disclosing s.
    Stasis hemostyptic s.
    Talbots iodine s.
    Trace disclosing s.

sol·vent
    Arti-Spot s.

So·no-Ex·plor·er

Sor·en·sen
    S. chisel

So·tos
    S. syndrome

sound
    affricative s.

space
    apical s.
    buccal s.
    closure s.
    cricothyroid s.
    Czermak's s's
    s's in dentin
    escapement s's
    freeway s.

space *(continued)*
    globular s's of Czermak
    interarch s.
    interdental s.
    interglobular s's (of Owen)
    interocclusal s.
    interproximal s.
    interproximate s.
    interradicular s.
    leeway s.
    Nance's leeway s.
    pharyngeal s.
    pharyngomaxillary s.
    primate s.
    proximal s.
    proximate s.
    pterygomandibular s.
    relief s.
    retromylohyoid s.
    retropharyngeal s.
    septal s.
    subgingival s.
    submandibular s.
    submaxillary s.
    thyrohyal s.

spac·er

spa·ti·um *pl.* spa·tia
    spatia interglobularia

spat·u·la

spat·u·late

spat·u·la·tion

spat·u·la·tor

Spec·tra-A strip

Spec·tra-F strip

Spec·tra-Points

Spec·tra-Sys·tem den·tal im·plant

spec·trum *pl.* spec·tra
    facio-auriculo-vertebral s.
    hyperthermia-induced s. of defects

spec·trum *(continued)*
    oromandibular-limb hypogenesis s. (mandibular hypodontia)

Spec·trum por·ce·lain

Spee
    reverse curve of S.
    S's curve
    S's curvature

speed·bond·ing

Speed lin·er

Spen·cer
    S. scissors

sphinc·ter
    s. oris

spill·way
    axial s.
    interdental s.
    occlusal s.

spin·dle
    enamel s's

spine
    mental s., external

spi·ra·my·cin

splint
    abutment s.
    acrylic s.
    acrylic resin bite-guard s.
    advancement s.
    anchor s.
    Angle's s.
    Asch s.
    biodegradable s.
    bite s.
    buccal s.
    cap s.
    Carter's intranasal s.
    cast bar s.
    compressive s.
    compressive facial s.
    continuous clasp s.
    copper band–acrylic s.

splint *(continued)*
    cross arch bar s.
    Denver s.
    diagnostic s.
    Doyle Airway S's
    Elbrecht s.
    Essig-type s.
    external fixed temporary s.
    fenestrated s.
    fixed s.
    fixed partial denture s.
    fixed permanent s.
    fracture s.
    Friedman s.
    Gilmer's s.
    Gunning's s.
    Hammond's s.
    implant surgical s.
    inlay s.
    interdental s.
    internal fixed temporary s.
    interocclusal s.
    Jones' nasal s.
    Kazanjian's s.
    Kingsley s.
    labial s.
    labiolingual s.
    lingual s.
    lingual arch wire s.
    maxillary s.
    molded s.
    nasal fracture s.
    occlusal s.
    one-piece Gunning s.
    onlay s.
    passive s's
    permanent s.
    polyglycolide s.
    pressure s.
    provisional s.
    removable permanent s.
    removable temporary s.
    temporary s.
    two-piece Gunning s.
splint·ing
    cross arch s.
    Essig-type s.

split·ting
    sagittal s. of mandible
spon·dy·li·tis
    ankylosing s.

sponge
    absorbable gelatin s.
    Banker's s.
    Bernays' s.
    cotton s.
    exodontia s.
    fibrin s.
    gelatin s.
    Nu Gauze s.
    Syngauze s.
    Topper s.
    Zobec s.

spoon
    s. excavator

spray
    Endo Ice refrigerant s.
    ethyl chloride s.

spread·er
    Endoteck s.
    finger s.
    root canal filling s.

spring
    alignment s.
    auxiliary s.
    Begg uprighting s.
    bow s.
    canine retraction s.
    closed s.
    Coffin s.
    coil s.
    finger s.
    free-end s.
    helical s.
    Kesling s.
    loop s.
    open s.
    paddle s.
    s. rate
    retraction s.
    separating s.
    split acrylic s.

spring *(continued)*
    uprighting s.
    Z s.

Spring White 10 whit·en·ing gel

sprue
    s. base
    s. pin

spur
    cementum s.
    enamel s.

squa·ma *pl.*squa·mae
    occipital s.

squa·mous

SSO
    sagittal split osteotomy

SSRO
    sagittal split ramus osteotomy

S.S. White (S.S.W.) clamp

S.S. White (S.S.W.) new fill·ing por·ce·lain

S.S. White (S.S.W.) pulp test·er

Sta·bi·lex at·tach·ment

sta·bil·i·ty
    denture s.
    dimensional s.
    occlusal s.

sta·bil·iza·tion
    Osteo-Loc endodontic s.

sta·bi·li·zer
    endodontic s.

Sta·bi·lok den·tal pin

Staf·ne
    S. defect

stage
    bell s.
    bud s.

stage *(continued)*
    cap s.
    preeruptive s.
    ugly duckling s.

stain
    Gomoramine methenamine silver (GMS) s's
    Masson's trichrome s.
    Minute S.
    periodic acid–Schiff (PAS) s.

stain·ing
    s. of teeth - extrinsic tetracycline s.

stamp
    cusp s.

Stand·al·loy

stan·dard
    Holdaway cephalometric s's
    Legan and Burstone cephalometric s's

Stan-Gard flu·o·ride gel

Staph·y·lo·coc·cus
    S. aureus
    S. epidermidis

staph·y·lo·coc·cus *pl.* staph·y·lo·coc·ci

Stark
    S. classification (for cleft palate)

Star·lite Om·ni-AT bur

Star·ret wire gauge

Star root ca·nal file

Sta·sis he·mo·styp·tic so·lu·tion

Stat BR bite reg·is·tra·tion ma·te·ri·al

State Board of Den·tal Ex·am·i·ners

State Board of Den·tist·ry

Sta-Tic im·pres·sion ma·te·ri·al

Sta·tus com·pos·ite res·in

STE
subperiosteal tissue
expander

steel
stainless s.

Steele
S's facing

Stei·ger
S's attachment
S's connector
S's joint
S.-Boitel attachment
S.-Boitel bar

Stei·glitz
S. pliers

Stein·er
S. analysis

Stein·häus·er plates

Stein·häus·er screws

Stein·häus·er Ti·ta·ni·um
Bone Plate Sys·tem

Stein·mann
S. pin

Ste·no
canal of S.
duct of S.

Sten·sen
S's canal
S's duct

stent
circumoral s.
drainage s.
labial periodontal s.
occlusal s.
pedodontic s.
periodontal s.
trismus s.

ster·i·li·za·tion
dry heat s.

Steri-Oss im·plant

Stern
S. attachment
S. G/A attachment
S. gingival latch
attachment
S. G/L attachment
S. stress-breaker
S. stress-breaker
attachment
S. stress-breaker unit

Stern·gold 1 gold al·loy

Stern·gold 2 gold al·loy

Stern·gold 3 gold al·loy

Stern·gold 5 gold al·loy

Stern·gold B gold al·loy

Stern·gold Bridg·ette In·lay

Stern·gold G-43 no·ble metal
al·loy

Stern·gold In·lay

Stern·gold S gold al·loy

Stern·gold Su·per·cast gold al·
loy

Ste·vens
S.-Johnson syndrome

stick
bite s.
compound tracing s.
mouth s.

stick-lac

Stick·ler
S. syndrome

Stie·glitz
S. fragment and root
forceps

Still·man
S's cleft

Still·man *(continued)*
    S's method of
      toothbrushing
    S's technique

Stim-U-Dent

stim·u·la·tor
    Bimler s.

Stim·u·la·tor ar·tic·u·la·tor

stip·pling
    gingival s.

sto·mat·ic

sto·ma·ti·tis *pl.* sto·ma·tit·i·
  des
    contact s.
    denture s.
    s. nicotina
    nicotine s.
    recurrent aphthous s.
    Vincent's s.

sto·ma·tog·nath·ic

sto·ma·tog·ra·phy

sto·ma·to·log·i·cal

sto·ma·tol·o·gist

sto·ma·tol·o·gy

sto·ma·to·plas·tic

sto·ma·to·plas·ty

sto·ma·to·scope

stone
    APL dental s.
    Arkansas s.
    black s.
    Blue Die Stone dental s.
    Brownie dental s.
    Class I s.
    Class II s.
    composite fine s.
    composite point s.
    cup s.
    Denstone dental s.
    dental s.

stone *(continued)*
    diamond s.
    die s.
    Diekeen dental s.
    Die Stone dental s.
    Dura-Green dental s.
    Dura-White dental s.
    Duroc dental s.
    flat s.
    Fuji Rock dental s.
    Glasstone dental s.
    gray s.
    gray-green s.
    Greenie dental s.
    improved s.
    Indic Die Stone dental s.
    Lab Stone dental s.
    mounted s.
    pulp s.
    red s.
    salivary s.
    Silky Rock dental s.
    Snap-Stone dental s.
    Supergreenie dental s.
    Supra Stone dental s.
    Tru-Stone dental s.
    Vel Mix dental s.
    wheel s.
    White Arkansas s.

stop
    centric s.
    incisal s.
    Krueger s.
    occlusal s.

stop·ping
    temporary s.

Stout
    S. continuous wiring
    S. wiring

strain
    compressive s.
    maximum principal s.
    minimum principal s.
    tensile s.

strap
  lingual s.
  palatal s.

Stra·to·sphere al·loy

stra·tum *pl.* stra·ta
  s. adamantinum
  s. basale
  s. corneum
  s. eboris
  s. germinativum
  s. granulosum
  s. intermedium
  s. spinosum

Streiff
  Hallermann-S. syndrome

strength
  compressive s.
  shear bond s.
  tensile s.
  transverse s.

Strep·to·coc·cus
  S. mitis
  S. mutans
  S. salivarius
  S. sanguis
  S. viridans

strep·to·coc·cus *pl.* strep·to·coc·ci
  alpha s.
  -hemolytic s.

strep·to·my·cin

stress
  axial s.
  s. equalizer
  lateral s.
  mises tensile s.
  occlusal s.

stress-break·er
  complete s.-b.
  Crismani s.-b.
  hinger s.-b.
  partial s.-b.
  Stern s.-b.

stria *pl.* striae
  Retzius' parallel striae
  Schreger's striae

strip
  abrasive s.
  alumox gapped s.
  gapped s.
  lightning metal s.
  linen s.
  Proflex scaling s.
  Spectra-A s.
  Spectra-F s.
  Suture S's
  zirconium gapped s.

stripe
  s's of Retzius

strip·min·ing

struc·ture
  denture-supporting s's

study
  Burlington growth s.

strut
  primary implant
    substructure s.
  secondary implant
    substructure s.

Sturd·i·cast al·loy

Sturge
  S.-Weber anomalad

sub·den·tal

sub·gin·gi·val

Sub·li·maze

sub·lux·a·tion
  atlantoaxial s.

sub·man·dib·u·lar

sub·max·il·la

sub·max·il·lary

sub·peri·os·te·al

sub·pul·pal

sub·stance
    adamantine s. of tooth
    interprismatic s.
    intertubular s. of tooth
    ivory s. of tooth
    proper s. of tooth

sub·stan·tia *pl.* sub·stan·tiae
    s. adamantina dentis
    s. eburnea dentis
    s. intertubularis dentis
    s. ossea dentis

sub·sti·tute
    dentin s.
    tin foil s.

sub·struc·ture
    implant s.

Suc·cess·Fil en·do·don·tic ob·tu·ra·tion sys·tem

Suc·cess·Fil gut·ta per·cha

Su·gar greater palatine s. of maxilla·man
    S. file
    S. Nipro nippers

sul·ci

sul·cus *pl.* sul·ci
    alveolabial s.
    alveolingual s.
    alveolobuccal s.
    s. colli mandibulae
    gingival s.
    s. gingivalis
    gingivobuccal s.
    gingivolingual s.
    greater palatine s.
    greater palatine s. of
        maxilla
    greater palatine s. of
        palatine bone
    labiodental s.
    lingual s.
    mandibular s.
    median s. of tongue
    s. medianus linguae
    mentolabial s.

sul·cus *(continued)*
    s. mentolabialis
    mylohyoid s. of mandible
    s. mylohyoideus
        mandibulae
    nasolabial s.
    s. nasolabialis
    palatine sulci of maxilla
    sulci palatini maxillae
    s. palatinus major maxillae
    s. palatinus major ossis
        palatini
    terminal s. of tongue
    s. terminalis linguae
    s. of tongue

sul·fate
    aluminum s.

Sul·li·van
    S. scissors

Sul·pak re·trac·tion cord

Sun·cast al·loy

Sun-Schein re·stor·a·tive

Su·per·Bite bite reg·is·tra·tion
    paste

Su·per·Body hy·dro·col·loid

su·per·erup·tion

Su·per·gel im·pres·sion ma·te·ri·al

Su·per·green·ie den·tal stone

Su·per·ox·ol bleach·ing agent

Su·per·paste im·pres·sion
    paste

Su·per Rub·ber im·pres·sion
    ma·te·ri·al

Su·per·sil im·pres·sion ma·te·ri·al

Su·per Snap buff disks

Su·per Snap pol·ish·ing sys·tem

Su·per Soft soft acryl·ic res·in

su·per·struc·ture
    implant s.

sup·port
    abutment s.
    cast s.
    fixed s.
    free s.
    multiple abutment s.
    restrained s.
    rugae s.
    tooth s.

sup·pu·ra·tion
    alveodental s.

su·pra·bulge

su·pra·clu·sion

su·pra·oc·clu·sion

Su·pra Stone Mix den·tal stone

su·pra·ver·sion

sur·face
    alveolar s. of maxilla
    anterior s.
    axial s.
    balancing occlusal s.
    basal s.
    buccal s.
    contact s.
    distal s.
    facial s.
    foundation s.
    impression s.
    incisal s.
    labial s.
    lateral s.
    lingual s.
    masticatory s.
    medial s.
    mesial s.
    morsal s's
    occlusal s., working
    occlusal s. of teeth
    oral s.
    parietal s. of parietal bone

sur·face *(continued)*
    polished s.
    polished s. of denture
    posterior s.
    proximal s.
    proximate s.
    subocclusal s.
    vestibular s.

Sur·flex F im·pres·sion ma·te·ri·al

sur·gery
    ambulatory s.
    combined jaw s.
    dental s.
    dentoalveolar s.
    dentofacial s.
    implant s.
    maxillofacial s.
    maxillofacial cosmetic s.
    mucogingival s.
    oral s.
    oral and maxillofacial s.
    orthognathic s.
    orthognathic mandibular s.
    periodontal s.
    preprosthetic s.
    reconstructive s.
    salvage s.
    segmental s.
    TMJ s.

Sur·gi·cel

Sur·gi·dent im·pres·sion ma·te·ri·al

sur·vey·ing

sur·vey·or
    dental s.
    Jelenko s.
    Ney s.
    Ney dental s.
    Williams s.

sus·pen·sion
    Adams s.

Sus·tain HA-bio·in·te·grat·ed den·tal im·plant sys·tem

Su·ter·a·loy amal·gam al·loy

su·tur·al

su·ture
    absorbable s.
    anchor s.
    braided Dacron s.
    braided silk s.
    catgut s.
    chromic s.
    chromic gut s's
    continuous sling s. type I
    continuous sling s. type II
    Dexon s.
    Ethicon s.
    harelip s.
    horizontal mattress s.
    incisive s.
    midface s.
    nonabsorbable s.
    O-Polydioxanone s.
      (O-PDS)
    palatine s., anterior
    palatine s., median
    palatine s., middle
    palatine s., posterior
    palatine s., transverse
    palato-ethmoidal s.
    palatomaxillary s.
    polyglycolic acid s.
    premaxillary s.
    Prolene s.
    silk s's
    sling s.
    vertical mattress s.
    Vicryl s.

Su·ture Strips

Su·zanne
    S's gland

Sved
    S. appliance therapy
    S.-type appliance

swage

swag·er

swal·low
    infantile s.

sweat·ing
    gustatory s.

Swede-Vent den·tal im·plant

swell·ing
    lingual s.

Sy·bra·loy al·loy

sym·phy·sis *pl.* sym·phy·ses
    s. mandibulae
    mandibular s.
    s. menti

Syn·cote amal·gam car·ri·er

syn·drome (see also under
    disease)
    Aarskog s.
    Aase s.
    achondrogenesis s's
    acquired immune
      deficiency s. (AIDS)
    acquired immunodeficiency
      s. (AIDS)
    Adams-Oliver s.
    aging face s.
    Albright's s.
    Angelman s.
    Antley-Bixler s.
    Apert's s.
    Ascher s.
    auriculotemporal s.
    autosomal recessive
      hypohidrotic ectodermal
      dysplasia s.
    basal cell nevus s.
    Beals's.
    Beckwith-Wiedemann s.
    Behçet's s.
    Binder s.
    Bloom s.
    Brody's s.
    burning mouth s.
    Caffey's s.
    Carpenter s.
    cat-eye s.

syn·drome *(continued)*
cerebrocostomandibular s.
cerebro-oculo-facio-skeletal s.
CHILD s.
chondrodysplasia punctata s.
Cockayne's s.
Coffin-Lowry s.
Coffin-Siris s.
Cohen's s.
combination s.
Costen's s.
Cowden's s.
CREST s.
Cross s.
Crouzon s.
de Lange's s.
DIC (disseminated intravascular coagulation) s.
disseminated intravascular coagulation s.
distal arthrogryposis s.
distichiasis-lymphedema s.
Down s.
Dubowitz s.
dyskeratosis congenita s.
Eagle's s.
Eagle-like s.
EEC s.
Ehlers-Danlos s.
Escobar s.
Fabry s.
femoral hypoplasia–unusual facies s.
fibrodysplasia ossificans progressiva s.
fragile X s.
Fraser s.
Freeman-Sheldon s.
Frey's s.
Gardner's s.
generalized gangliosidosis s., type I
Goltz s.
Gorlin's s.

syn·drome *(continued)*
Hajdu-Cheney s.
Hallermann-Streiff s.
Hand-Schüller-Christian s.
Hay-Wells s.
Hecht s.
Heerfordt's s.
homocystinuria s.
Horner's s.
Hunter's s.
Hurler s.
Hurler-Scheie compound s.
hypohidrotic ectodermal dysplasia s.
incontinentia pigmenti s.
Jaffe-Lichtenstein s.
Job's s.
Johnson-Blizzard s.
Killian and Teschler-Nicola s.
Langer-Giedion s.
large face s.
Larsen's s.
Lenz-Majewski hyperostosis s.
leprechaunism s.
Leroy I–cell s.
lethal multiple pterygium s.
Letterer-Siwe s.
Levy-Hollister s.
long face s.
Lowe s.
Marfan s.
Maroteaux-Lamy mucopolysaccharidosis s.
Marshall's s.
Marshall-Smith s.
Meckel-Gruber s.
Melkersson-Rosenthal s.
Melnick-Needles s.
Mietens s.
Mikulicz's s.
Miller s.
Miller-Dieker s.
Mohr s.
Morquio s.
multiple lentigines s.

syn·drome *(continued)*
  multiple neuroma s.
  multiple synostosis s.
  Nager s.
  Neu-Laxova s.
  nevoid basal cell carcinoma
    s.
  Noonan's s.
  numb chin s.
  s. of the numb chin
  obstructive sleep apnea s.
    (OSAS)
  oculodentodigital s.
  Opitz s.
  oral-facial-digital s.
  orofaciodigital s.
  osteogenesis imperfecta s.
  otopalatodigital s.
  otopalatodigital s., type II
  4p⁻ s.
  5p⁻ s.
  9p⁻ s.
  18p⁻ s.
  pachyonychia congenita s.
  pain dysfunction s.
  Pallister-Hall s.
  Papillon-Lef43evre s.
  partial trisomy 10q s.
  Peutz-Jeghers s.
  Pfeiffer's s.
  Plummer-Vinson s.
  popliteal web s.
  Prader-Willi s.
  progeria s.
  13q s.
  18q⁻ s.
  radial aplasia–
    thrombocytopenia s.
  Rapp-Hodgkin ectodermal
    dysplasia s.
  Reiter's s.
  Rieger's s.
  Roberts-SC phocomelia s.
  Robinow's s.
  Rothmund-Thomson s.
  Rubinstein-Taybi s.
  Russell-Silver s.
  Ruvalcaba's s.

syn·drome *(continued)*
  Saethre-Chotzen s.
  Sanfilippo's s.
  Scheie's s.
  Schinzel-Giedion s.
  Schwartz-Jampel s.
  Seckel's s.
  Senter s.
  short face s.
  Shprintzen's s.
  Sjögren's s.
  Sjögren-Larsson s.
  Smith-Lemli-Opitz s.
  Sotos's.
  Stevens-Johnson s.
  Stickler s.
  temporomandibular
    dysfunction s.
  temporomandibular joint s.
  Treacher Collins s.
  tricho-dento-osseus s.
  trichorhinophalangeal s.
  triploidy s.
  trisomy 4p s.
  trisomy 8 s.
  trisomy 9 mosaic s.
  trisomy 9p s.
  trisomy 13 s.
  trisomy 18 s.
  trisomy 20p s.
  tuberous sclerosis s.
  Van der Woude's s.
  Waardenburg's s.
  Weaver s.
  Weill-Marchesani s.
  Werner s.
  Williams s.
  XO s.
  XXXX s.
  XXXXY s.
  XYY s.
  Zellweger s.

Syn·gauze sponge

syn·os·to·sis
  bicoronal s.

sy·no·vi·al

syno·vi·tis
  villonodular s.

syn·tax·is

Syn·thes AO/ASIF sys·tem

Syn·thes dy·nam·ic com·pres·
  sion plate

syph·i·lis

sy·ringe
  air s.
  Aquafix irrigating s's
  chip s.
  Cook-Waite aspirating s.
  dental s.
  endodontic s.
  endodontic irrigating s.
  Endovage s.
  Henke-Ject s.
  hydrocolloid s.
  intraligamental s.
  Luer:Lok s.
  Miltex N-Tralig
    Intraligamentary
    Anesthesia S.
  Monoject s.
  pressure s.
  Pulpdent s.
  self-aspirating s.
  Technitouch aspirating s.
  water s.

sys·tem
  All-Bond 2 bonding s.
  All-Bond 2 Dental
    Adhesive S.
  Amalgam Bond bonding s.
  AO-THORP reconstruction
    s.
  arcon articulator-facebow
    s.
  Arnett-TMP rigid fixation
    s.
  Automix Computerized
    Mixing S.
  bonding s.
  Bondlite bonding s.
  Bosker TMI s.

sys·tem *(continued)*
  Brånemark Implant S.
  Castmatic-S titanium
    casting s.
  Cerec CAD/CAM s.
  Cervident bonding s.
  Clearfil Photo-Bond
    bonding s.
  Composhape finishing s.
  Concise Orthodontic
    Bonding S.
  Concise White Sealant S.
  Cosmic Bond bonding s.
  Cure-Thru Wedge S.
  dental adhesive s.
  Dentatus anchorage s.
  dentinal s.
  dentin bonding s.
  Dewey classification s.
  Dumbach Titanium Mesh
    S.
  Dumbach titanium plating
    s.
  endosteal implant s.
  Enhance finishing and
    polishing s.
  Espe Rocatec-S.
  Filpin s.
  FluoroCore Core Build-up
    S.
  Gluma bonding s.
  Gluma 3 Step bonding s.
  HiLite bleaching s.
  IMZ Hex Implant S.
  Interpore Hex Implant S.
  ITI Dental Implant S.
  ITI non-submerged dental
    implant s.
  K4 anchor s.
  Kerr composite finishing s.
  Kerr endopost s.
  Kurer anchor s.
  Löe index s.
  Luhr maxillofacial s.
  Luhr microfixation s.
  masticatory s.
  Micro Plus titanium
    plating s.

sys·tem *(continued)*
    microfixation s.
    Mini Würzburg titanium
      plating s.
    Mirage-Bond bonding s.
    Mirage Plus bonding s.
    MPS diamond polishing s.
    non–self-tapping s.
    Osseodont Dental Implant
      S.
    Osteo-Loc Plate Form S.
    Osteo-Loc Root Form S.
    Para Post s.
    Paulus Titanium Chin
      Plate S.
    Paulus titanium plating s.
    Pertac Universal Bond
      bonding s.
    Photobond bonding s.
    Power Bond bonding s.
    Prisma Universal Bond 2
      bonding s.
    Prisma Universal Bond 3
      bonding s.
    Prisma Universal bonding
      s.
    Radix Anchor s.
    Salzburg titanium plating
      s.
    Scotchbond bonding s.
    Scotchbond 2 bonding s.
    self-tapping s.
    Shofu Super Snap disk s.
    Silicoater silica coating s.
    Sof-Lex finishing and
      polishing s.
    Sof-Lex Pop-On disk s.
    Steinhäuser Titanium
      Bone Plate S.
    Steinhäuser titanium
      plating s.
    stomatognathic s.
    SuccessFil endodontic
      obturation s.

sys·tem *(continued)*
    Super Snap polishing s.
    Sustain HA-biointegrated
      dental implant s.
    Synthes AO/ASIF s.
    Tenure bonding s.
    Therabite jaw motion
      rehabilitation s.
    Threadmate s.
    3-D titanium plating s.
    Titanium Plasma Sprayed
      Screw S.
    titanium plating s.
    TPS implant s.
    Triad II light cured s.
    Triad VLC s.
    Triad VLC (visible
      light–cured) resin s.
    Two-Striper MPS polishing
      s.
    Vintage/Opal Porcelain S.
    visible light–cured (VLC)
      resin s.
    visible light–curing (VLC)
      s.
    VisionPlus cosmetic
      imaging s.
    Würzburg fracture s.
    Würzburg reconstruction s.
    Würzburg Titanium
      Fracture S.
    Würzburg Titanium
      Mandibular
      Reconstruction S.
    Würzburg Titanium Mini
      Bone Plate S.
    Würzburg Titanium
      Orthognathic Implant S.
    Würzburg titanium plating
      s.
    XR Bond bonding s.
    XR Primer/XR Bond
      bonding s.

tab
    bite-wing t.

tab·let
    Red Cote disclosing t.
    Reveal disclosing t.

Tach-E-Z at·tach·ment

Tach-E-Z re·tain·er

Tag·gard
    T's compressed-gas casting
        machine
    T's machine
    T's method

tal·am·pi·cil·lin

tal·on

tang

tan·ta·lum

tape
    dental t.
    floss t.

tar·nish

tat·too

tau·ro·don·tism

Tay·bi
    Rubinstein-T. syndrome

Tay·lor
    Semken-T. forceps
    T. scaler

T-band ma·trix

T-bar el·e·va·tor

T bar of Ka·zan·jian

TC
    tungsten carbide

TC-A carv·er

TC-B carv·er

TC-C carv·er

TC-D carv·er

TC-E carv·er

TCP im·plants

TEAM den·tist·ry

teas·er
    Davis root tip t.

tech·ne·ti·um
    t. Tc 99m methylene
        diphosphonate

tech·nique
    Akinosi t.
    angle bisection t.
    aseptic t.
    banding t.
    Barkann's t.
    barrier t.
    Bass' t.
    bead t.
    Begg t.
    bisecting angle t.
    bisection of angle t.
    Bowles t.
    Box's t.
    bulk t.
    bulk pack t.
    Burstone's arch t.
    calibrated angle t.
    capping t's
    Caspersson t.
    channel shoulder pin t.
    Charters' t.
    compensation t.
    continuous-gum t.
    controlled water added t.
    copper tube t.
    CSP (channel shoulder
        pin) t.
    differential force t.
    direct t.
    double pour t.

tech·nique *(continued)*
    dry field t.
    dual impression t.
    Eames' t.
    edgewise t.
    filling bead t.
    filling brush t.
    filling flow t.
    fluorescent antibody t.
    half-mouth t.
    heat casting t.
    high heat casting t.
    impression t.
    indirect t.
    injection-molding t.
    investment hygroscopic
      expansion t.
    investment thermal
      expansion t.
    Johnston-Callahan
      diffusion t.
    Jorgensen t.
    labiolingual t.
    light round wire t.
    lip switch t.
    lost wax t.
    Nealon's t.
    nonpressure t.
    one-phase subperiosteal
      implant t.
    one-pour t.
    open flap t.
    parallel t.
    paralleling t.
    porcelain cervical contact
      and single bake t's
    porcelain cervical ditching
      t.
    pressure t.
    push-back t.
    ribbon arch t.
    right-angle t.
    single pour t.
    sinus lift t.
    Stillman's t.
    subperiosteal implant one-
      phase t.
    "switch stick" t.

tech·nique *(continued)*
    syringeless hydrocolloid
      impression t.
    two-pour t.
    vector t.
    V-Y t.
    wash t.
    washed field t.
    wax pattern thermal
      expansion t.

Tech·ni·touch as·pi·rat·ing sy·
  ringe

teeth

Tef·lon

Tef·lon FEP

Tef·lon poly·tet·ra·flu·o·ro·
  eth·yl·ene (PTFE)

tel·an·gi·ec·ta·sia
    hereditary hemorrhagic t.

te·maz·e·pam

Tem-Pac Cool-Jaw

Tem·pak ce·ment

Temp-Bond ce·ment

Temp-Bond NE ce·ment

Temp-Ca·nal paste

Tem·pit fill·ing and seal ma·
  te·ri·al

tem·plate
    Bolton t.
    occlusal t.
    scalloped endosseous t.
    surgical t.
    wax t.

tem·po·ral

tem·po·ro·man·dib·u·lar

tem·po·ro·max·il·lary

Tem·rex ce·ment

TEN
toxic epidermal necrolysis

Te·na·cin ce·ment

ten·sion
interfacial surface t.

tens·om·e·ter

Ten·ure bond·ing sys·tem

Tesch·ler-Ni·co·la
Killian and T.-N.
syndrome

Tes·si·er
T. forceps

test
cold pulp vitality t.
electric pulp t.
electric pulp vitality t.
fluorescein t.
hardness t.
heat pulp vitality t.
Jones 1 t.
Jones 2 t.
penetration t.
pulp t.:
pulp vitality t.
quantitative precipitation
t.
Schirmer's t.
scleroscope t.:
shear t.
thermal discrimination t.
thermal pulp vitality t.
tooth mobility t.
transillumination pulp
vitality t.
uniaxial pullout t's
Von Frey t.

test·er
electric pulp t.
high frequency pulp t.
low frequency pulp t.
Olsen stiffness t.
Ritter t.
S.S.W. pulp t.
stiffness t.

test·er *(continued)*
torque t.

test·ing
electrical pulp t.
electronic pulp t.

tet·ra·cy·cline

TG/O chis·el

thal·as·se·mia

the·co·dont

the·o·ry
acidogenic t.
Begg's t.
dimer t.
Moss functional matrix t.
proteolysis-chelation t.

Ther·a·bite jaw mo·tion re·ha·
bil·i·ta·tion sys·tem

Ther·a·bite per·son·al ex·er·
cis·er

Ther·a·Pac·er

ther·a·peu·tic
accepted dental t.
provisionally accepted
dental t.
unaccepted dental t.

ther·a·peu·tics

ther·a·py
anxiolytic t.
endodontic t.
hyperbaric oxygen t.
myofunctional t.
occlusal bite plate t.
pulp canal t.
root canal t.
Sved appliance t.

Ther·ma·fil

Ther·mo·dent

ther·mo·plas·tic

ther·mo·set·ting

thim·ble

Thin-Flex disk

Thi·o·kol

Thi·o·kol rub·ber im·pres·sion

thio·pen·tal so·di·um

Thixo-Gel flu·o·ride gel

Thomp·son
    T. dowel

Thom·son
    Rothmund-T. syndrome

thread
    elastomeric t.

Thread·mate sys·tem

Thread Timed Trans·fer Pins

3-D
    three-dimensional

3-DBRP
    three-dimensional,
        bendable reconstruction
        plate

throm·bo·cy·to·pe·nic

throm·bo·sis
    cavernous t.
    cavernous sinus t.

thrush

thrust
    tongue t.

thy·ro·glos·sal

thy·roid
    lingual t.

tic
    t. douloureux

ti·car·cil·lin

Ti·co·ni·um hid·den-lock den·ture

Ti·co·ni·um Or·tho·don·tic Wire

Ti-Core core ma·te·ri·al

time
    amalgam setting t.

Time·line base/lin·er

Ti·Mesh bone screws

Ti·Mesh Soft·plate

Ti·Mesh ti·ta·ni·um mesh

tin
    t. oxide

tin·foil

tip
    interdental t.
    t. of tongue

tip·ping
    t. of cusp
    labiolingual t.

tis·sue
    adipose t.
    hematopoietic t.
    metastases to the soft oral
        t.
    periodontal t.

ti·ta·ni·um
    t. nitride

Ti·ta·ni·um Plas·ma Sprayed
    Screw Sys·tem

TMD
    temporomandibular
        disorder
    temporomandibular
        dysfunction

TMJ
    temporomandibular joint

TMJ Con·dy·lar Pros·the·sis

TMJ Fos·sa Em·i·nence Pros·the·sis

TMJS
    temporomandibular joint
        syndrome

TMS
　　thread mate system

TMS Link Plus re·ten·tion pin

TMS pin

to·bac·co
　　smokeless t.

to·bra·my·cin

Tomes
　　T. fiber
　　T. fibril
　　granular layer of T.
　　T. process

to·mog·ra·phy
　　computed t.
　　cross-sectional spiral t.
　　three-dimensional
　　　　computed t.

ton·er
　　F.I.T.T. functional
　　　　impression tissue t.
　　ectopic oral t's

tongue
　　adherent t.
　　amyloid t.
　　antibiotic t.
　　baked t.
　　bald t.
　　beefy t.
　　bifid t.
　　black t.
　　black hairy t.
　　blue t.
　　burning t.
　　cardinal t.
　　cerebriform t.
　　choreic t.
　　cleft t.
　　coated t.
　　cobble-stone t.
　　crescent t.
　　crocodile t.
　　dotted t.
　　double t.
　　earthy t.

tongue *(continued)*
　　encrusted t.
　　fern leaf t.
　　filmy t.
　　fissured t.
　　flat t.
　　frog t.
　　furred t.
　　furrowed t.
　　geographic t.
　　glazed t.
　　grooved t.
　　hairy t.
　　hobnail t.
　　lobulated t.
　　magenta t.
　　mappy t.
　　parrot t.
　　plicated t.
　　raspberry t.
　　raw-beef t.
　　Sandwith's bald t.
　　scrotal t.
　　smokers' t.
　　smooth t.
　　split t.
　　stippled t.
　　sulcated t.
　　timber t.
　　trombone t.
　　white t.
　　wooden t.
　　wrinkled t.

ton·sil
　　adenoid t.
　　buried t.
　　eustachian t.
　　faucial t.
　　Gerlach's t.
　　lingual t.
　　nasopharyngeal t.
　　palatine t.
　　pharyngeal t.
　　submerged t.

ton·sil·la *pl.* ton·sil·lae
　　t. adenoidea
　　t. lingualis

ton·sil·la *(continued)*
    t. palatina
    t. pharyngea
    t. pharyngealis

ton·sil·lar

ton·sil·li·tis

ton·sil·lo·li·thi·a·sis

tooth *pl.* teeth
    abutment t.
    accessional teeth
    accessory t.
    anatomic teeth
    anchor t.
    ankylosed t.
    anterior teeth
    artificial t.
    auditory teeth of Huschke
    baby teeth
    bicuspid teeth
    buccal teeth
    canine teeth
    cheek teeth
    conical t.
    connate t.
    corner t.
    Corti's auditory t.
    cross-bite teeth
    cross-pin teeth
    cuspid teeth
    cuspless t.
    cutting t.
    dead t.
    deciduous teeth
    diatoric teeth
    drifting t.
    embedded t.
    eye t.
    Fournier teeth
    fused teeth
    geminate t.
    Goslee t.
    green t.
    hag teeth
    hereditary brown
      opalescent t.
    Horner's teeth

tooth *(continued)*
    Hutchinson's teeth
    hutchinsonian t.
    impacted t.
    incisor teeth
    intruded t.
    labial teeth
    malacotic teeth
    malposed t.
    mandibular teeth
    maxillary teeth
    metal insert t.
    migrating t.
    milk t.
    molar teeth
    Moon's teeth
    morsal teeth
    mottled teeth
    mulberry t.
    multicuspid t.
    natal t.
    neonatal t.
    nonanatomic teeth
    nonsyndrome
      supernumerary teeth
    nonvital t.
    notched t.
    peg t.
    peg-shaped t.
    pegtop t.
    permanent teeth
    pink t. of Mummery
    pinless teeth
    posterior teeth
    predeciduous t.
    premature teeth
    premolar teeth
    primary teeth
    pulpless t.
    rake teeth
    rational teeth
    rootless teeth
    rotated t.
    sclerotic teeth
    screwdriver teeth
    shell t.
    snaggle t.
    stomach t.

tooth *(continued)*
    straight-pin teeth
    submerged t.
    succedaneous teeth
    successional teeth
    superior teeth
    supernumerary teeth
    supplemental teeth
    syphilitic t.
    temporary teeth
    Trubyte Bioblend Denture
      teeth
    tube teeth
    Turner's t.
    unerupted t.
    vital teeth
    wandering t.
    wisdom t.
    wolf t.
    zero degree teeth

tooth-borne

tooth·brush
    Bass' t.
    electric t.
    interproximal t.
    multituft t.
    powered t.

tooth·brush·ing
    Bass' method of t.
    Charters' method of t.
    crevicular method of t.
    Fones' method of t.
    maxillofacial and
      facioproximal surface t.
    maxillopalatal and
      palatoproximal surface t.
    modified Stillman's method
      of t.
    occlusal surface t.
    physiologic method of t.
    scrub-brush method of t.
    Stillman's method of t.

Tooth Col·or In·di·ca·tor

Tooth·keep·er

tooth·paste

To·pex 00:60 flu·o·ride gel

To·pex pro·phy·lax·is paste

Top·i·cale an·es·thet·ic gel

Top·i·cale li·quid

To·pi·nard
    T's angle
    T's line

Top·per sponge

To·ra·loy

To·ri·tron

torque
    lingual root t.

torqu·ing

tor·sion

tor·si·ver·sion

to·rus *pl.* to·ri
    mandibular t.
    t. mandibularis
    palatal t.
    t. palatinus

Town·er
    T. scaler

tox·o·plas·mo·sis

TPS im·plant sys·tem

Trace dis·clos·ing so·lu·tion

trac·er
    arrow-point t.
    needle-point t.
    stylus t.

trac·ing
    arrow-point t.
    cephalometric t.
    cephalometric prediction t.
    extraoral t.
    Gothic arch t.
    intraoral t.
    needle-point t.
    prediction t's
    stylus t.

trac·tion
    external t.
    intermaxillary t.
    internal t.
    maxillomandibular t.
    maxillomandibular elastic
        t.

tran·ex·am·ic acid

trans·acet·y·la·tion

trans·acet·y·la·tion

trans·fer
    hinge-axis facebow t.
    microvascular tissue t.

trans·la·tion

trans·la·tor
    FMA t.

trans·lu·cen·cy

trans·lu·cent

trans·pal·a·tal

trans·plan·ta·tion
    tooth t.

trau·ma *pl.* trau·mas, trau·ma·ta
    maxillofacial t.
    occlusal t.
    t. from occlusion
    t. from oral sex
    potential t.
    toothbrush t.

trau·mat·ic

tray
    acrylic resin t.
    alloplastic t.
    bite registration t.
    Check-Bite t.
    impression t.
    mesh t's
    Rim-Lock impression t.
    Rite Bite t.
    stock t's

tray *(continued)*
    Triad VLC acrylic
        impression t.
    triple t.

Trea·cher Col·lins
    T.C. syndrome

treat·ment
    age hardening heat t.
    P.T. pulp t.
    radio-frequency glow
        discharge t.

treph·i·na·tion
    dental t.

Tre·po·ne·ma
    T. denticola
    T. pallidum
    T. vincenti

Tri·ad 2000 light cur·ing unit

Tri·ad gel

Tri·ad II light cured sys·tem

Tri·ad pro·vi·sion·al ma·te·ri·al

Tri·ad VLC acryl·ic im·pres·sion tray

Tri·ad VLC bond·ing agent

Tri·ad VLC di·rect re·line ma·te·ri·al

Tri·ad VLC res·in sys·tem

Tri·ad VLC sys·tem

tri·am·cin·o·lone

tri·an·gle
    Assézat's t.
    Bolton t.
    Bonwill t.
    facial t.
    frontal t.
    palatal t.
    retromandibular t.
    retromolar t.
    Tweed t.

tri·a·zo·lam

tri·cus·pid

trid·y·mite

tri·gem·i·nal

tri·gone

tri·gon·id

tri·meth·y·lene

trim·mer
    acrylic t.
    gingival margin t. (GMT)
    margin t.
    model t.
    plaster t.
    proximal t.
    wax t.

trim·ming

trip·le-an·gle

trip·o·li

tri·stea·rin

trit·ur·a·ble

trit·ur·ate

trit·ur·a·tion
    manual t.
    mechanical t.
    mortar and pestle t.

trit·ur·a·tor
    mechanical t.
    Silamat t.
    Vari-Mix t.

Tro·po·sphere al·loy

Tru·byte Bio·blend Den·ture
  Teeth

True
    T's separator

Tru·lin·er den·ture re·line

Tru-Soft den·ture re·line

Tru-Stone den·tal stone

Tru·wax base plate wax

try-in

T-type ream·er

tube
    Brook airway-resuscitating
      t.
    buccal t.
    end t.
    horizontal t.
    nasotracheal t.
    vertical t.

tu·ber *pl.* tu·bers, tu·be·ra
    external t. of Henle
    mental t.

tu·ber·cle
    Carabelli t.
    condyloid t.
    dental t.
    genial t.
    mental t.
    mental t., external
    mental t. of mandible
    pterygoid t.

tu·ber·cu·lo·sis

tu·ber·cu·lum *pl.* tu·ber·cu·la
    t. coronae
    t. geniale

tu·be·ros·i·ty
    masseteric t.
    t. of maxilla
    pterygoid t. of mandible

tu·ber·ous

Tu·bin·ger
    T. implant

Tu·bli-Seal

tu·bule
    dental t's
    dentinal t's

Tuck·er
    T. bougie

tuft
    enamel t's

tu·mor
    acinar cell t.
    acinic cell t.
    adenomatoid t.
    adenomatoid odontogenic
        t.
    basaloid mixed t.
    benign mixed t.
    calcifying epithelial
        odontogenic t.
    carcinoma ex mixed t.
    central giant cell t.
    clear cell odontogenic t.
    desmoid t.
    giant cell t. of bone
    granular cell t.
    malignant mixed t.
    malignant nerve t.
    malignant nerve sheath t.
    malignant triton t.
    melanotic neuroectodermal
        t.
    melanotic neuroectodermal
        t. of infancy
    metastatic t's to the jaws

tu·mor *(continued)*
    mucoepidermoid t.
    odontogenic t.
    Pindborg t.
    plasma cell t.
    primitive neuroectodermal
        t.
    salivary gland t.
    spindle cell t.
    squamous odontogenic t.
    Warthin's t.

tur·bi·nec·to·my

Tur·ner
    T's teeth

Tweed
    T. pliers
    T. triangle

Two·Point·One XE la·ser

Two-Strip·er MPS pol·ish·ing
    sys·tem

Ty·lok-Plus ce·ment

ty·po·dont

Ty·tin al·loy

Ty·tin com·pos·ite res·in

ula·ga·nac·te·sis

ulal·gia

ulat·ro·phy
    afunctional u.
    atrophic u.
    calcic u.
    ischemic u.
    traumatic u.

ul·cer
    recurrent aphthous u.
      (RAU)
    traumatic u's

ul·cer·a·tion
    herpetiform u's

ul·cer·a·tive

ulec·to·my

uli·tis

ulot·o·my

ulo·trip·sis

Ul·tra·Gold al·loy

un·der·cut

un·der·struc·ture

uni·cus·pid

uni·cus·pi·date

uni·cys·tic

Uni-Etch

Uni·file

Uni·gauge han·dle

Uni·Jel im·pres·sion ma·te·ri·al

Uni-Pro pro·phy paste

Uni·son al·loy

unit
    Acri-Dense 3 curing u.
    AutoMix mixing u.
    Capmix mixing u.
    Cavitron u.
    C & L u.
    Crismani combined u.
    Dalbo extracoronal u.
    Dalbo stud u.
    dental u.
    Dolder bar u.
    intraoral curing u's
    Mixomat mixing u.
    Pressomatic u.
    Silamat mixing u.
    Stern stress-breaker u.
    Triad 2000 light curing u.

Uni·ver·si·ty of Min·ne·so·ta re·trac·tor

Uni·ver·si·ty of Wash·ing·ton rub·ber dam clamp for·ceps

UPPP
    uvulopalatopharyngoplasty

up·right·ing

U/P root ca·nal ce·ment

uvu·la *pl.* uvu·lae
    bifid u.

uvu·lo·pal·a·to·phar·yn·go·plas·ty (UPPP)

vac·cine
anticaries v.

Va·cu·dent

Val·iant Ph.D. al·loy

Val·iant Snap-Set al·loy

Val·i·um

Val·mid

val·ue
Harvold standard v's

Va·na·dium

van·co·my·cin

Van·cou·ver mi·cro·sto·mia or·tho·sis

Van der Woude
Van der W. syndrome

var·i·cel·la

var·i·cos·i·ties

Vari·Glass glass ion·o·mer

Vari-Mix tri·tu·ra·tor

Vari-Mix III Amal·ga·ma·tor

Var·nal cav·i·ty var·nish

var·nish
Caulk v.
cavity v.
copal cavity v.
Copalite v.
mastic v.
periodontal v.
rosin v.
Varnal cavity v.

vault

Veau
V. classification (for cleft palate)

Vehe
V. carver

vein
jugular v.

Vel·ban

Vel·cro

Vel·foam

Vel Mix den·tal stone

Velv·al·loy amal·gam al·loy

ve·neer
full v.

ver·a·pam·il hy·dro·chlo·ride

Veri·best 22 Kt in·lay

Ver·mil·lion
Greene-V. index

Ver·nier
V. caliper

Ver·rill
V. sign

ver·ru·ca *pl.* ver·ru·cae
v. vulgaris

ver·ru·ci·form

ver·ru·cous

Ver·sa·tile hy·dro·col·loid

Ver·sed

ves·tib·u·lar

ves·ti·bule
buccal v.
labial v.
v. of mouth

ves·tib·u·lo·plas·ty
mandibular v.
split-thickness skin graft v.

VHN
  Vickers hardness number

vi·bra·tion
  v. condensation

vi·bra·tor

Vib·rio
  V. succinogenes

Vick·ers
  V. hardness indenter point
  V. hardness number
    (VHN)
  V. hardness scale
  V. hardness test
  V. indenter
  V. indenter point
  V. scale

Vi·co·din ES

Vi·cryl su·ture

Vin·cent
  Plaut-V. infection
  V's gingivitis
  V's infection
  V's stomatitis

Vin·son
  Plummer-V. syndrome

Vin·tage/Opal Por·ce·lain Sys·
  tem

vi·nyl
  v. acetate
  v. chloride
  v. polysiloxane

Vir·chow
  V's line

Vis·co-gel tis·sue con·di·tion·
  er and lin·er

Vi·sio-Dis·pers re·stor·a·tive

Vi·sio-Fil com·pos·ite res·in

Vi·sio-Fil re·stor·a·tive

Vi·sion·Plus cos·met·ic imag·
  ing sys·tem

Vi·sio-Seal pit and fis·sure seal
  ·ant

Vis·ta·ril

Vi·ta·blocs Mark II

Vi·ta·dur-N

vi·tal·i·ty
  pulp v.

Vi·tal·li·um al·loy

Vi·ta-Lu·min shade de·sig·na·
  tion

Vi·tre·bond base/lin·er

VLC
  visible light–cured
  visible-light-curing

VLC res·in

Vogt
  V's angle
  V's point
  V.-Hueter point

Von Frey
  Von F. test

von Lan·gen·beck
  von L's bipedicle
    mucoperiosteal flap
  von L. palatoplasty
  von L. procedure

von Wil·le·brand
  von W's disease

VPS (vinyl polysiloxane) im·
  pres·sion ma·te·ri·al

vul·ca·nize

Vul-Cryl·ic scrap·er

vul·ga·ris

Vy·cor glass

Waar·den·burg
  W's syndrome

Wachs
  W. paste

wa·fer
  bite w.
  Coprwax bite w.

Wag·ner
  W. scissors

Walk·er
  W. appliance
  W. articulator

Wall
  W. waxing instrument

wall
  axial w.
  cavity w.
  enamel w.
  gingival w.
  incisal w.
  peripheral w.
  pocket w.
  pulpal w.
  subpulpal w.

Wal·sham
  W. forceps

Wal·ther
  W's duct

wan·der·ing
  pathologic tooth w.

W-arch

War·thin
  W's tumor

wax
  adhesive w.
  Allcezon base plate w.
  barnsdahl w.
  base plate w.

wax *(continued)*
  baseplate w.
  bees w.
  w. bite
  bite w.
  bleached w.
  blockout w.
  bone w.
  boxing w.
  Brazil w.
  w. burn-out
  candelilla w.
  carding w.
  carnauba w.
  casting w.
  ceresin w.
  corrective w.
  dental w.
  dental inlay casting w.
  earth w.
  w. expansion
  fluxed w.
  fossil w.
  Horsley's w.
  impression w.
  inlay casting w.
  inlay pattern w.
  Japan w.
  Kerr hard w.
  Kerr regular w.
  microcrystalline w.
  mineral w.
  model denture w.
  montan w.
  natural w.
  NeoWax baseplate w.
  ouricury w.
  paraffin w.
  pattern w.
  Peck's purple hard w.
  plant w.
  processing w.
  set-up w.
  sticky w.

wax *(continued)*
    sumac w.
    synthetic w.
    Truwax base plate w.
    try-in w.
    utility w.
    vegetable w.
    white w.
    yellow w.

wax·ing

wax·ing up

wax out

wax-up
    diagnostic w.-u.
    esthetic w.-u.

wear
    interproximal w.

Weav·er
    W. syndrome

Web·er
    Sturge-W. anomalad
    W.-Fergusson incision

We·del·staedt
    W. chisel

WED·JETS den·tal dam cord

We·ge·ner
    W's granulomatosis

Weil
    W's basal layer
    W's basal zone

Weill
    W.-Marchesani syndrome

Weis·bach
    W's angle

Wel·cher
    W's angle

well
    amalgam w.

Wells
    Hay-W. syndrome

Wer·ner
    W's syndrome

West
    W. periosteal elevator

Wes·ton
    W. crown

Whar·ton
    submaxillary duct of W.
    W's duct

wheel
    bristle w.
    buffing w.
    Burlew w.
    Carborundum w.
    Ceramisté w.
    chamois w.
    cotton w.
    diamond w.
    felt w.
    grinding w.
    leather w.
    polishing w.
    rag w.
    rubber w.
    wire w.

Whip-Mix ar·tic·u·la·tor

Whip-Mix Die-Rock

Whip-Mix Mi·cro·stone

Whip-Mix Quick·stone

Whip-Mix Silky-Rock

White·side
    W. scaler

wi·den·er
    orifice w.

Wid·man
    modified W. flap
    W. flap

Wiede·mann
    Beckwith-W. syndrome

Wie·der
    W. retractor

Wig-L-Bug amal·ga·ma·tor

Wilde
    W's incision

Wil·li
    Prader-W. syndrome

Wil·liams
    Fox-W. probe
    Neurohr-W. rest shoe
    W. periodontal probe
    W. probe
    W. round probe
    W. surveyor
    W. syndrome

Wilms
    aniridia–W. tumor
        association

wire
    arch w.
    arch w., ideal
    bending w.
    brass w.
    buccal stabilizing w.
    circummandibular w.
    diagnostic w.
    ideal arch w.
    Jelenko super w.
    Kirschner w.
    labial w.
    ligature w.
    measuring w.
    Mowrey 12% w.
    Mowrey No. 1 w.
    orthodontic w.
    Risdon's w.
    separating w.
    skeletal suspension w's
    stainless steel w.
    suspension w's
    Ticonium Orthodontic W.
    twin w.
    wrought w.

wir·ing
    Baudens w.
    Black w.
    Buck w.

wir·ing *(continued)*
    circumferential w.
    circumpalatal w.
    circumzygomatic w.
    continuous loop w.
    craniofacial suspension w.
    Gilmer w.
    interosseous w.
    mandibular w.
    Ivy loop w.
    perialveolar w.
    piriform aperture w.
    Robert w.
    Stout w.
    Stout continuous w.
    suspension w.
    transalveolar w.

Wits
    W. analysis

Wiz·ard frame

Wo·li·nel·la
    W. recta

Wood
    Crile-W. needle holder

Wood·side
    W. activator

Wood·son
    W. elevator
    W. filling instrument

Wood·ward
    W. elevator

W-plasty

W/P (wa·ter-pow·der) ra·tio

Wurz·burg
    W. screws

Würz·burg frac·ture sys·tem

Würz·burg re·con·struc·tion

Würz·burg ti·ta·ni·um con·dy·
    lar plate

Würz·burg Ti·ta·ni·um Frac·
    ture Sys·tem

Würz·burg Ti·ta·ni·um Man·
   dib·u·lar Re·con·struc·tion
   Sys·tem

Würz·burg Ti·ta·ni·um Mini
   Bone Plate Sys·tem

Würz·burg Ti·ta·ni·um Or·
   tho·gnath·ic Im·plant Sys·
   tem

Würz·burg ti·ta·ni·um plat·
   ing sys·tem

Xan·ax

xan·tho·fi·bro·ma

xan·tho·gran·u·lo·ma

xan·tho·ma
    verruciform x.

Xan·to·pren

X-bite

xe·ro·sto·mia

XR Bond bond·ing sys·tem

XR Prim·er/XR Bond bond·ing
    sys·tem

Xy·lo·caine

Y ax·is

Y-clo·sure

yoke
    alveolar y's of mandible
    alveolar y's of maxilla

Young
    Y. frame

Young·er
    Y. scaler
    Y.-Goode curet

Y plate

Zan·tac

Za·ro·sen de·sen·si·tiz·er

Zell·weg·er
    Z. syndrome

Zest An·chor sys·tem at·tach·ment

Zest im·plant an·chors

zinc
    z. oxide
    z. oxide powder
    z. oxyphosphate
    z. phenolsulfonate

Zir·cate pro·phy paste

Zir·con F pro·phy paste

zir·co·ni·um

Zir·ox·ide pro·phy paste

Zo·bec sponge

ZOE
    zinc oxide–eugenol

ZOE-B&T base and tem·po·rary fill·ing ma·te·ri·al

ZOE ce·ment

ZOE im·pres·sion paste

zone
    apical z.
    cervical z.
    contact area z.
    coronal z.
    dentofacial z.
    neutral z.
    occlusal z.
    rugae z.
    z's of Schreger
    Weil's basal z.

Z-plasty
    double Z-p.
    Furlow double Z-p.

Z100 re·stor·a·tive

Z100 re·stor·a·tive spher·i·cal hy·brid

Z spring

zy·go·ma

zy·go·mat·i·co·max·il·lary